CLINICAL EPIDEMIOLOGY

MONOGRAPHS IN EPIDEMIOLOGY AND BIOSTATISTICS

Edited by Michael G. Marmot, Jonathan M. Samet,
David Savitz, Martin P. Vessey

Monographs in Epidemiology and Biostatistics
Volume 36

CLINICAL EPIDEMIOLOGY

The Study of the Outcome of Illness

Third Edition

Noel S. Weiss

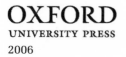

UNIVERSITY PRESS

2006

OXFORD
UNIVERSITY PRESS

Oxford University Press, Inc., publishes works that further
Oxford University's objective of excellence
in research, scholarship, and education.

Oxford   New York
Auckland   Cape Town   Dar es Salaam   Hong Kong   Karachi
Kuala Lumpur   Madrid   Melbourne   Mexico City   Nairobi
New Delhi   Shanghai   Taipei   Toronto

With offices in
Argentina   Austria   Brazil   Chile   Czech Republic   France   Greece
Guatemala   Hungary   Italy   Japan   Poland   Portugal   Singapore
South Korea   Switzerland   Thailand   Turkey   Ukraine   Vietnam

Published by Oxford University Press, Inc.
198 Madison Avenue, New York, New York 10016

www.oup.com

Oxford is a registered trademark of Oxford University Press

Library of Congress Cataloging-in-Publication Data
Weiss, Noel S., 1943–
   Clinical epidemiology : the study of the outcome of illness / Noel S. Weiss. — 3rd ed.
      p. ; cm. — (Monographs in epidemiology and biostatistics ; v. 36)
   Includes bibliographical references and index.
   ISBN-13 978-0-19-530523-4
   ISBN 0-19-530523-X
   1. Clinical epidemiology.   I. Title.   II. Series.
   [DNLM: 1. Epidemiologic Methods. 2. Biometry. 3. Treatment Outcome.   W1 MO567LT v.36
2006 / WA 950 W431c 2006]
RA652.2.C55W45 2006
614.4—dc22   2005031889

9 8 7 6 5 4 3 2 1
Printed in the United States of America
on acid-free paper

Series Introduction

Monographs in Epidemiology and Biostatistics

The Monographs in Epidemiology and Biostatistics are intended to promote the development of the field of epidemiology and its applications. Through a continued series of publications, the monographs will advance the methodologic foundation of the field, as well as more specific areas of epidemiologic inquiry. The monographs are intended to be useful for both students and epidemiologic researchers and practitioners. There are three broad themes for the series.

1. Monographs on the epidemiology of specific topics of health or disease or specific methodologic areas that should serve as reference material and course texts for graduate training. As new themes coalesce in the field and as old themes evolve, these monographs should provide a resource that captures the essential features of the topic and that are useful for organizing courses.
2. Monographs on disciplines setting the foundation for epidemiology that are needed to place the field of epidemiology in context. These topics include the underpinning from philosophy and history and from sociology and behavioral sciences, as well as the place of the discipline in regard to ethics and regulatory and policy issues. By definition, epidemiology is an applied discipline, and those applications point to issues worthy of careful examination.
3. Monographs that address the interface of epidemiology with other disciplines. Epidemiology relates with increasing frequency and in-

tensity to clinical sciences, basic science, and social sciences. Monographs are called for that can explore those interfaces and provide texts to help educate epidemiologists who wish to understand how to become engaged with other disciplines, and they are also useful for those from other disciplines who seek to engage with epidemiology and epidemiologists.

To serve these purposes, the series will engage the leading thinkers and researchers as authors so that readers can continue to trust the series to provide a modern, thoughtful, and readable perspective on the most pressing topics in epidemiology.

Preface to the Third Edition

The first edition of this book was published in 1986, the second in 1996. Now that 2006 is upon us, is a third edition of *Clinical Epidemiology* called for? Other than the passing of another decade, there are several reasons that I chose to answer this question in the affirmative:

1. The intervening years saw the design, conduct, and publication of a number of clinical epidemiologic studies that illustrated particularly well some of the methods and principles that had been described in the earlier editions. I wanted to incorporate these as examples.

2. Developments in the field, particularly in the area of randomized controlled trials, made me feel that the second edition was now incomplete. In particular, the topic of meta-analysis—unmentioned in the earlier editions—today assumes a great deal of importance in the evaluation of the consequences of treatment. The desire to deal with this topic in the appropriate depth led me to invite a colleague with substantial expertise in meta-analysis, Peter Cummings, to take the lead in composing an entire chapter devoted to it.

A number of colleagues and students at the University of Washington—Peter Cummings, Tom Koepsell, Bruce Psaty, Loren Dalrymple, Wendy Langeberg, Kathryn Adeney, Annette Adams, Nancy Morden, and Ian de Boer—reviewed and commented on drafts of individual chapters, and the book has benefited from their efforts.

Ideally, the provision of health care would judiciously employ effective tests and treatments that have a minimum of untoward consequences. To the extent that this book helps some investigators to design and analyze their evaluations of tests or treatments to produce valid results, or leads some readers of clinical epidemiologic research to better interpret the findings of that research, my goal in writing it will have been accomplished.

Contents

CLINICAL EPIDEMIOLOGY

1

Clinical Epidemiology

What It Is and How It Is Used

Let's say that among your patients is a middle-aged man with intermittent claudication and that his symptoms have been increasing in severity over the last several years. His blood sugar level is normal, but he has a long history of cigarette smoking. The results of the physical examination are normal except for the absence of pulses in his legs. The systolic blood pressure measured in the dorsalis pedis artery is only 70% of that measured in the brachial artery. Should he be advised to undergo ultrasound and/or arteriographic evaluation and an operation for any surgically correctable lesions?

Among the questions that need to be addressed before making such a recommendation are the following:

1. What is the expected progression of symptoms and expected longevity in such a patient in the absence of surgical intervention?
2. To what extent are the available diagnostic tests capable of (a) identifying remediable lesions, (b) not producing false-positive results, and (c) not producing adverse effects?
3. What is the likelihood (short- and long-term) that surgery will relieve symptoms or prevent progression without causing complications?

Clinical epidemiology is the area of research that attempts to provide answers to these sorts of questions.

Epidemiology is the study of variation in the occurrence of disease and of the reasons for that variation. It first entails making *observations* of the occurrence of illness or injury in individuals and of those characteristics

3

that distinguish affected from unaffected persons. This process is followed by the formation of *inferences* as to which of these characteristics, or other, unmeasured ones, play a role in causing the disease.

Clinical epidemiology is defined here in a parallel way. It is the study of variation in the *outcome* of illness and the reasons for that variation. The modus operandi is similar as well. First, observations are made on the fate of ill persons—who recovers, who worsens, who develops complications—and what characterizes those with different fates. Second, inferences are drawn regarding the particular characteristics of the patients or their care that were responsible for these differences in outcome.

For many conditions, the most important determinants of outcome are diagnostic and therapeutic interventions. Because research in clinical epidemiology attempts to quantify the importance of particular interventions relative to others or to none at all, the results have direct applications for providers of health care.

To illustrate the questions that epidemiology and clinical epidemiology try to answer, let's return to the topic of intermittent claudication. Epidemiologic studies would make observations pertinent to the etiologies of the symptom and its underlying pathology: Cigarette smokers and nonsmokers might be contrasted regarding the prevalence of claudication. If these studies indicated a strong relationship, perhaps one that increased with the amount and recency of smoking, and if nonepidemiologic evidence were compatible with a deleterious effect of cigarette smoking on the peripheral arteries, then an inference of cause and effect could be drawn.

Clinical epidemiology, however, focuses on the consequences of the condition and the care given for it. Thus observations might be made: on untreated patients with claudication regarding the rate of change in symptoms; on similar patients undergoing sonography and arteriography to determine the prevalence of surgically correctable lesions; and on still others who undergo surgery to assess the change in symptoms and/or physical signs. These studies would lead to inferences as to the role of the diagnostic tests and surgery in the management of patients with claudication. The results of the studies would address questions such as the following: To what extent is there improvement of symptoms and signs as a result of these procedures? Alternatively, to what extent could any observed favorable outcomes be attributed to spontaneous regression of disease or to selection for surgical therapy of patients destined to have favorable outcomes? If testing followed by surgery is believed to produce improvements, what proportion of the patients undergoing these tests was helped? By how much? Quantitative answers are necessary, for they will have to be balanced against the costs and hazards of sonography/arteriography and surgery.

The term "illness" is part of the definition of clinical epidemiology, and it is used here in a broader sense than "disease," which often refers to a particular set of anatomic or physiologic abnormalities. Illness may, for example, denote only a symptom that causes a patient to seek care or a physical sign detected by a provider of care. Because a large part of the utility of research in clinical epidemiology lies in its evaluation of the work of providers of health care, I use the term "illness" to refer to any reason that people have for seeking the services of such a provider. The methods of clinical epidemiology operate in the same way whether they are applied to persons seeking care for health maintenance, for a specific symptom or sign, or for a disease.

Clinical Epidemiology in Relation to Clinical Decision Making

Our decision to perform a test on a patient requires, as a first step, an affirmative answer to the following questions:

1. Do the test results improve our ability to predict the occurrence of an outcome we are seeking to prevent? For example, do the results of fecal occult blood screening discriminate between patients who are and are not likely to die from colorectal cancer?
2. Taking into account the results of the test, are we able to treat patients in such a way as to decrease the likelihood of the outcome and/or reduce the occurrence of adverse effects of treatment? Does treatment of patients with cancers detected through fecal occult blood screening offer an advantage over treatment later in the course of illness, once signs or symptoms have developed?

If the answer is "yes" to both questions, we must quantify the health benefits we expect to achieve. Next, we need to determine whether the monetary costs related to testing are an "acceptable" price to pay. In the example we are considering, once we have estimated the reduced probability of death and disability from colorectal cancer in patients offered testing for fecal occult blood, it is necessary to ask whether that reduction is large enough to justify the cost of the test and the cost of evaluation of false-positive results that will occur.

In deciding whether to administer a treatment, much the same type of thinking takes place. It is necessary to weigh the estimated overall benefit of the treatment against that provided by alternative interventions and to determine whether the cost of treatment can be justified.

A key aim of research in clinical epidemiology is to document accurately the health consequences of employing a test or administering a therapy. Deciding whether interventions that lead to favorable consequences should be used—those that can be "justified" given their costs—is the task of the health care provider and his or her patient, with increasingly strong guidance from society (Eddy, 1991a,b).

When making decisions concerning public health interventions, each society must ration the resources it commits to reducing the probability of illness and death among its members. We are willing to pay just so much for road safety, for example. It is probable that additional highway dividers or railroad bridges would prevent some injuries and an occasional accidental death, but in many instances we are unable to "afford" them. Or perhaps we may believe that installation of a highly trained emergency medical service in a town of 10,000 persons could prevent the death of 1 person who develops cardiac arrest each year, but it is likely that in many towns of this size, the expense of such a program exceeds what the populace is willing to pay.

Because society is responsible for the overwhelming majority of health care expenditures, the wishes of society should play a role in determining the allocation of *individual* health care expenses, as well. Though a provider of health care is committed to doing everything possible to promote a patient's health, the range of what is possible should be delineated by those who will pay the bill. Thus there are instances in which a health care provider, conscious of society's needs, will make recommendations or take actions that fall short of those that he or she would implement if resources for health care were unlimited. Such a provider realizes that these resources *are* limited— what is consumed for one purpose is not available for others. The goal of the health care provider, then, is to use these finite resources in the most efficient way. For example, a provider might do a Pap smear every 3 years rather than more frequently in women already screened negative several times, not because this approach is adequate to prevent all mortality from cervical cancer in such patients but because it is a reasonably inexpensive way to prevent *most* of it.

> *Example:* In patients with acute chest pain, several clinical charac-
> teristics have been identified that are correlated with the presence of
> myocardial infarction. A group of investigators (Fineberg et al., 1984)
> attempted to assess the economic and health implications of two types
> of acute care in patients with chest pain who were in a "low" risk group
> (probability of myocardial infarction less than 1 in 20): (a) admission
> to a coronary care unit versus (b) admission to an "intermediate" care
> unit (i.e., one that would permit electrocardiographic monitoring and
> the administration of antiarrhythmic medications but not intensive
> nursing care). They estimated that there would be a small excess of
> deaths from ventricular fibrillation and complete heart block in the
> group placed in intermediate care. Nonetheless, they concluded that
> "patients who have a low risk for myocardial infarction would be ap-
> propriate candidates for admission to an 'intermediate' care unit, since
> the provision of the facilities of a coronary care unit to all low risk
> patients would cost an estimated additional $2 million per life saved."

Sadly, during the first part of the twenty-first century in some parts of the world, financial constraints are such that even some relatively inexpen- sive health interventions are too costly to provide to individual patients. For example, in Uganda the national coordinator of a project devoted to the prevention of mother-to-child HIV transmission cited cost as one justification for his government's inability to provide infant formula to HIV-positive mothers. Rhetorically, he asked, "Can we afford it? Are we justified to add infant formula when our health centers don't have even the basic antenatal care drugs such as folic acid? In a resource-constrained system we have to be pragmatic and do what is possible" (Wendo, 2003).

At present, resources in North America and Europe may not be so tightly constrained as those in Uganda, but most health care providers and patients are well aware of the constraints nonetheless. Tests and treatments are increasingly judged not only on their efficacy but also on efficacy per unit cost. Note, in the following excerpts from an article in a 2002 issue of *The New England Journal of Medicine* (Gaspoz et al., 2002), the contrast between the positive findings regarding the efficacy of the new drug cited in the first paragraph and the negative clinical recommendations for use of that drug that are made in the second paragraph.

> Clopidogrel, a thienopyridine derivative, was shown to reduce the relative risk of ischemic stroke, myocardial infarction, or death from vascular causes in patients with prior cardiovascular disease by 8.7 percent as compared with aspirin, and the addition of clopidogrel to aspirin for patients with acute coronary syndromes reduced the risk of death from cardiovascular causes, reinfarction, and stroke by 20 percent as compared with aspirin alone.
>
> Increased prescription of aspirin for secondary prevention of coronary heart disease is attractive from a cost-effectiveness perspective. Because clopidogrel is more costly, its incremental cost effectiveness is currently unattractive, unless its use is restricted to patients who are ineligible for aspirin.

Instruction in a formal method for considering both health benefits and monetary costs in medical decision making—decision analysis—can be found elsewhere (Petitti, 2000), along with examples of the application of this method to selected patient management issues.

References

Eddy DM. The individual vs. society: Is there a conflict? *JAMA* 1991a;265: 1446, 1449–1450.

Eddy DM The individual vs. society: Resolving the conflict. *JAMA* 1991b;265: 2399–2406.

Fineberg HV, Scadden D, Goldman I. Care of patients with a low probability of acute myocardial infarction: Cost effectiveness of alternatives to coronary-care-unit admission. *N Engl J Med* 1984;310:1301–1307.

Gaspoz J-M, Coxson PG, Goldman PA, et al. Cost effectiveness of aspirin, clopidogrel, or both for secondary prevention of coronary heart disease. *N Engl J Med* 2002;346:1800–1806.

Petitti, DB. *Meta-Analysis, Decision Analysis, and Cost Effectiveness Analysis: Methods for Quantitative Synthesis in Medicine.* Oxford, New York, 2000.

Wendo G. HIV-positive mothers in Uganda resort to breast feeding. *Lancet* 2003;362:542.

2

Diagnostic and Screening Tests

Measuring Their Ability to Predict Adverse Outcomes of Illness

Providers of health care perform tests on a patient largely to obtain information that will influence the management of that patient's care. If the test is done in response to a symptom, sign, or condition known to be present in the patient, it is referred to as a "diagnostic" test. Tests that are performed in the absence of symptoms or signs in order to identify illnesses at an early stage or to identify predictors of future illness are termed "screening" tests. When you as a provider choose to buy information in the form of the results of diagnostic or screening tests, you do so because you believe that the value of the information exceeds its price. The value of a test result depends both on its accuracy and on how important the result is in leading to action(s) that bear on the individual's well-being.

The accuracy of a test depends, in turn, on its reliability—the degree to which repeated measurements give the same result—and its validity—the degree to which it measures what it intends to. The following example introduces some measures of test validity:

Example: Although the majority of persons having an acute myocardial infarction experience chest pain, most persons with chest pain have another basis for their symptoms. Because of the potential lethality of a myocardial infarction, physicians hospitalize many patients with chest pain for a period of time until they are reasonably certain that a myocardial infarction has not occurred. In an attempt to avoid hospitalization for patients with chest pain who do not have an infarction, Goldman et al. (1982) sought to develop clinical criteria to better predict the presence of myocardial infarction. (For a general discussion of the uses of clinical criteria as a form of diagnostic test, see Wasson et al., 1985.) For all patients with chest pain who were seen in an emergency room over a period of several months, they obtained information on characteristics at the time the patient was first seen and on each patient's status 6–10 months later. To some extent, the presence of myocardial infarction—determined during hospitalization or the follow-up period by EKG changes, elevated serum levels of cardiac enzymes, or abnormalities on radionuclide testing—was predicted by an algorithm that considered EKG abnormalities present during the emergency room visit, the nature and duration of symptoms experienced at that time, and the patient's age. Persons classified as "positive" or "negative" according to the algorithm experienced a myocardial infarction as follows:

Table 2.1. Emergency Room Criteria for Infarction

	Myocardial infarction present		
	Yes	No	Total
Positive	50	91	141
Negative	5	211	216
Total	55	302	357

The validity of the clinical criteria (the "test") could be described in terms of the degree to which persons with and without the condition under study (myocardial infarction) are correctly categorized. So the percentage of persons with an infarction who tested positive by the clinical criteria—the "sensitivity" of the criteria—was $50/55 \times 100 = 90.0\%$. The percentage of persons without an infarction who were correctly categorized as negative by the criteria—the "specificity"—was $211/302 \times 100 = 69.9\%$.

Alternatively, the validity of the criteria could be expressed as the extent to which being categorized as positive or negative actually predicts the presence of a myocardial infarction. In this example, the percentage of persons who were deemed clinically positive and who were found to have an infarction—the predictive value of a positive test $(PV+)$—was $50/141 \times 100 = 35.5\%$. The percentage who were clinically negative and who truly had no infarction—the predictive value of a negative test $(PV-)$—was $211/216 \times 100 = 97.7\%$. These measures are summarized in Table 2.2.

Estimation of Predictive Value under Various Sampling Schemes

Obviously, having an understanding of the validity of the clinical criteria in predicting the presence of a myocardial infarction is only the first step in reaching a decision as to whether these criteria should be used in managing

Table 2.2.   Measures of the Validity of a Diagnostic or Screening Test

General				Example			
Test	Reference criterion					No	
criterion	Positive	Negative	Total		Infarction	infarction	Total
Positive	a	b	a + b	Positive	50	91	141
Negative	c	d	c + d	Negative	5	211	216
Total	a + c	b + d		Total	55	302	

Term	General	Example	Definition
a. Sensitivity	a/(a + c)	50/55 (90.9%)	Proportion of those with the condition who have a positive test
b. Specificity	d/(b + d)	211/302 (69.9%)	Proportion of those without the condition who have a negative test
c. Predictive value of a positive test (PV+)	a/(a + b)[a]	50/141 (35.5%)	Proportion of those with a positive test who have the condition
d. Predictive value of a negative test (PV−)	d(c +d)[a]	211/215 (97.7%)	Proportion of those with a negative test who do not have the condition

[a] Meaningful only if (a + c)/n represents the actual proportion of true positives in the relevant population. If this condition does not hold, the test's sensitivity and specificity must be augmented with other information to estimate the predictive values (see pp 12–15).

patients with chest pain. It is also necessary to take into account the relevant costs—of applying the criteria to individual patients, of hospitalizing a patient with chest pain, and of the morbidity and mortality from myocardial infarction—before an informed decision can be made. An outline of the consequences of the 2 options—hospitalization only for clinically positive patients versus hospitalization for all with chest pain—with respect to the frequency of morbidity and mortality resulting from myocardial infarction is presented in Figure 2.1.

Consider first the upper portion of Figure 2.1, which deals with the consequences of a policy of hospitalization only for patients with chest pain who are clinically "positive." Estimating the occurrence of death and disability in patients managed according to this policy requires, as a first step, estimation of the prevalence of infarction in those who are either clinically "positive" or "negative." In this example, the proportion of "positive" patients who have a myocardial infarction is 50/141 (i.e., the $PV+$). The proportion of "negative" patients who have an infarction is 5/216 (i.e., $1 - PV-$). Thus it is the $PV+$ and $PV-$ that we would like to estimate with particular accuracy from studies that evaluate the validity of a test. For this reason, we must be aware of some commonly used study designs from which it is *not* possible to calculate directly $PV+$ and/or $PV-$.

(1) A study of the validity of screening criteria for myocardial infarction might compare the known cases with a sample of noncases rather than with

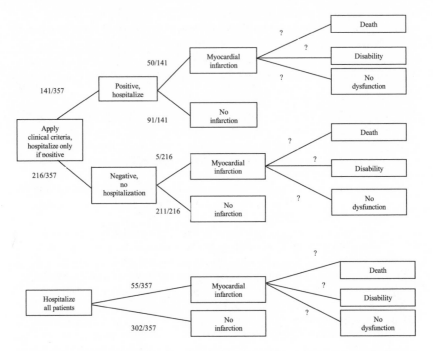

Figure 2.1 Death and disability associated with chest pain under two strategies for patient management.

the entire group of patients with chest pain who did not have an infarction. In the following example, equal numbers of noncases and cases have been chosen. If the proportion of screened-positive and screened-negative patients among noncases mirrors that of the total population of noncases—(91/302) x 55 = 17 falling in the positive group—the data would appear as follows:

Table 2.3

	Myocardial infarction		
Screening criteria	Yes	No	Total
Positive	50	17	67
Negative	5	38	43

Clearly, it would be incorrect to calculate $PV+$ as 50/67 or $PV-$ as 38/43. These calculations are strongly affected by the relative number of persons in the groups with and without infarction, and, in this example, these numbers have been arbitrarily set (1 control per 1 patient with infarction). However,

the sensitivity and specificity of the screening criteria can be accurately determined (each is calculated *within* the group of myocardial infarction cases
and noncases, respectively), and if the frequency of the condition that the
test seeks to identify can be estimated in patients to be tested, both predictive values can be estimated as well. A straightforward way of doing this is
as follows:

1. Pick, arbitrarily, a number representing the size of the total group
   that might be tested (or screened). Let's say you choose 10,000.
2. Multiply this number by the prevalence of the condition for which
   testing is being performed. Let's say you happen to know that the
   prevalence of myocardial infarction in patients seeking care for
   chest pain is 15.4% (i.e., the prevalence in the full study of 357
   patients). Thus, of the 10,000 patients, 1,540 would have an infarction and 8,460 would not.
3. a. Multiply the number of patients with the condition by the sensi-
      tivity of the test to determine the number of true positives.
   b. Multiply the number of patients without the condition by the
      specificity of the test to determine the number of true negatives.
4. By subtraction, determine the number of false negatives and false
   positives. In this example, there would be 140 false negatives (1,540
   − 1,400) and 2,615 false positives (8,460 − 5,845). The resulting table
   should look like this:

Table 2.4

	Myocardial infarction		
Clinical criteria	Yes	No	Total
Positive	1,540 × 50/55 = 1,400	2,615	4,015
Negative	140	8,460 × 38/55 = 5,845	5,985
Total	1,540	8,460	10,000

5. Calculate the *PV*+ and *PV*− from the numbers in the table:

$$PV+ = 1,400/(1,400 + 2,615) = 34.9\%$$

$$PV- = 5,845/(5,845 + 140) = 97.7\%$$

These values are identical (but for the errors due to rounding) to
those calculated from the entire group of 357 patients with chest
pain.

The *PV*+ also can be calculated using the following formula (Bayes's the-
orem):

$$PV+ = \frac{p(D)(sensitivity)}{p(D)(sensitivity) + 1 - p(D)(1 - specificity)}$$

$$PV+ = \frac{p(D)}{p(D) + \dfrac{1 - p(D)}{LR+}}$$

where $p(D)$ is the prevalence of the condition for which testing or screening is being performed and $LR+$, the likelihood ratio for a positive test, is sensitivity/ $(1 - \text{specificity})$. The $PV-$ can be calculated in a similar way:

$$PV- = \frac{p(D)}{1 - p(D) + [p(D)LR-]}$$

where $LR-$, the likelihood ratio for a negative test, is $(1 - \text{sensitivity}) / $ specificity. In the present example:

$$p(D) = 0.1541, 1 - p(D) = 0.8459$$

$$LR+ = \frac{50 \div 55}{38 \div 55} = 2.9412$$

$$LR- = \frac{1 - (50 \div 55)}{38 \div 55} = 0.1316$$

Thus

$$PV+ = \frac{0.1541}{0.1541 + \dfrac{1 - 0.1541}{2.9412}} = 0.349$$

and

$$PV- = \frac{0.8459}{0.8459 + (0.1541)(0.1316)} = 0.977.$$

In summary, the accurate estimation of $PV+$ and $PV-$ requires either (a) the use of a study population in which the frequency of the condition being tested for approximates that of the population in which the results are to be applied or (b) a knowledge of the frequency of the condition in the population in which the results are to be applied. The requirements underscore the influence of the frequency of the condition in the population being tested on the size of the predictive values and, ultimately, the influence of that frequency on the usefulness of the test in question. If a condition is uncommon, even a test that is highly sensitive and specific may produce a *PV+* that is quite low. The following table, constructed for a test with both sensitivity and specificity of 97%, illustrates this phenomenon:

Table 2.5.   Proportion of the Tested
Population with the Condition

Proportion	PV+	PV–
0.1	0.782	0.997
0.01	0.246	0.9997
0.001	0.031	0.99997
0.0001	0.003	0.999997

In this example, only when 10% of the persons receiving the test have the condition is *PV+* greater than 0.5. For a frequency of 1/1,000 or less, *PV+* is so low (≤ 0.031) that the test would probably not be useful for clinical or public health purposes. (It would be useful only if the cost of a false positive were exceedingly small compared with the benefit of identifying a true positive.) The *PV–* gradually approaches 1.0 with decreasing disease frequency and, compared with the *PV+*, exhibits little variation. However, keep in mind that even small changes in the *PV–* may be crucial in deciding whether or not a test should be used. For example, one reason that physicians might choose *not* to screen patients with chest pain for possible hospital admission is the not-so-small proportion of such patients who screen as negative and yet truly do have a myocardial infarction (2%–3%). For some physicians, this proportion might have to be reduced—perhaps by the development of yet more sensitive clinical criteria for the presence of a myocardial infarction— before they would be comfortable with a policy of admission only of selected patients with chest pain.

(2) The previous example dealt with studies in which the proportion of persons with and without the condition for which testing was done (e.g., myocardial infarction) did not reflect those of the population in which the results were to be applied (e.g., patients with chest pain admitted to an emergency department). Conversely, there are situations in which the criteria that determined which patients being studied did and did not receive the test differ from those used in the population in which the results are to be applied. For instance, suppose you are analyzing data from a second hospital emergency department that treated the same number of clinically positive patients as in the example in Table 2.1 but to which patients with very mild chest pain also came for evaluation. Instead of the ratio of positive to negative cases of 141/216 encountered in that example, perhaps the ratio now is 141/648. Assuming that the frequency of myocardial infarction among these 432 additional clinically negative cases were the same as among the original 216, the

data relating the clinical screening criteria to the occurrence of myocardial infarction would look like this:

Table 2.6

	Myocardial infarction		
Screening criteria	Yes	No	Total
Positive	50	91	141
Negative	15	633	648
Total	65	724	789

Though the sensitivity has decreased and the specificity has increased (to $633/724 = 0.86$) in comparison with the corresponding values in Table 2.2, the predictive values are the same as before ($PV+ = 50/141 = 0.355$; $PV- = 633/648 = 0.977$). Apparently all that has changed are the proportions of clinically positive and clinically negative patients.

But there is a possible pitfall here. Among persons with chest pain who are "negative" according to the clinical criteria decided on by the investigators, there will be a spectrum of severity. Those with the least pain may be the least likely to go to the emergency department and also the least likely to have an infarction. So, of the 432 additional clinically negative patients with chest pain coming to the second emergency department, there may be no patients with infarction rather than the 10 expected. In this particular scenario, both the specificity and the $PV-$ would be affected: $PV-$ would be $643/648 = 0.992$, a value higher than that obtained for the first emergency department, where the $PV-$ was $211/216 = 0.977$. (The $PV+$ will be unaffected by all of this, for it is based only on results in clinically positive individuals.) Thus, in order for a $PV-$ observed in a study population to be applied in a valid way in another population, it is necessary to consider the similarity of the 2 populations with respect to the types of patients that did and did not receive the test.

(3) If the patients with a condition or illness who are being studied are not typical of ill persons for whom the test is intended, with respect to the likelihood of a positive test result, neither the $PV+$ nor the $PV-$ can be estimated in a valid way. For example, if a fecal occult blood test were administered to symptomatic persons with colorectal cancer rather than to the asymptomatic population for whom it is meant to be administered for screening purposes, the calculated sensitivity would almost certainly be artificially high. It is probable that symptomatic patients have a relatively more advanced condition and would have a higher probability of having blood in their stool. Thus, even though the specificity of testing for fecal occult blood could be assessed accurately in this design—specificity is based solely on the results in noncases—the $PV+$ and $PV-$ would be falsely high.

Begg (1987) and Freedman (1987) provide examples of other situations in which estimation of the various measures of test validity may be biased.

Estimation of Predictive Value from Tests That Have the Potential to Do More Than Categorize Patients As Positive or Negative

The results of many tests are reported not as "positive" or "negative" but rather on a categorized or continuous scale. Persons are not measured as being "positive" for systolic hypertension; instead, their systolic blood pressure is assessed to the nearest millimeter of mercury. A test that requires interpretation (e.g., an X-ray or an EKG) can produce a result that is "intermediate" or "borderline" instead of simply positive or negative. Can the notion of predictive value be extended to cover test results that produce more than 2 possible outcomes?

The answer is "yes," if we are willing to settle for predictive values for a number of categories of test results that do not overtax the available data. For example, if we wish to estimate the predictive value of various levels of systolic blood pressure for the occurrence of stroke, we generally aggregate blood pressure levels into large enough groups—perhaps using intervals of 10 mm Hg—to get meaningful numbers of outcome events.

As an example, suppose that the algorithm developed in the study of clinical predictors of myocardial infarction (among patients with chest pain) could have subdivided the "positive" group into 2 categories—"strongly positive" and "borderline positive." Suppose that the following results were obtained:

Table 2.7

Test result	Myocardial infarction		
	Yes	No	Total
Strongly positive	38 (46.3%)	44 (53.7%)	82
Borderline positive	12 (20.3%)	47 (79.7%)	59
Negative	5 (2.3%)	211 (97.7%)	216
Total	55 (15.4%)	302 (84.6%)	357

Among persons who, based on their signs and symptoms, were "strongly positive," 46.3% actually had a myocardial infarction. The corresponding values for "borderline positive" and "negative" patients are 20.3% and 2.3%, respectively. Each of these values can be compared not only with one another but also with the unconditional probability of a myocardial infarction, that is, the overall probability that does not consider the results of the algorithm (55/357 = 15.4%). In the same way, the probability of *not* having a myocardial infarction can be calculated for the 3 possible categories the algorithm produced: 53.7%, 79.7%, and 97.7% for persons who were evaluated as strongly positive, borderline positive, and negative, respectively.

It may happen that, because of the way in which subjects were chosen for study, the ratio of persons with and without disease will not reflect the true ratio. As before, you may have chosen to compare the 55 patients who truly had a myocardial infarction with the 55 other patients with chest pain who ultimately were found to have no infarction. Even if the test being considered yields more than a dichotomous result, it is possible to estimate predictive values. Let's say the following data were obtained:

Table 2.8

Test result	Myocardial infarction	
	Yes	No
Strongly positive	38 (0.6909)[a]	8 (0.1455)
Borderline positive	12 (0.2182)	9 (0.1636)
Negative	5 (0.0909)	38 (0.6909)
Total	55 (1.00)	55 (1.00)

[a] Numbers in parentheses are the proportions of patients with or without a myocardial infarction with a test result in each of the three categories. For example, 38/55 = 0.6909.

The probability that a patient with a given result actually has an infarction can be calculated as follows:

$$PV+ = \frac{p(D)}{p(D) + \dfrac{1 - p(D)}{LR+}}$$

where $p(D)$ = probability of the disease in the population in which the test would be applied (typically, this is estimated from other sources), and $LR+$ = sensitivity / (1 – specificity). Let's assume our estimate for $p(D)$ is 0.154 (the value that was obtained in the full study of 357 patients). For the category "strongly positive," the $LR+$ is 0.6909/0.1455 = 4.750. Thus the chances that a patient in that category has an infarction are:

$$\frac{0.154}{0.154 + \dfrac{1 - 0.154}{4.750}} = 0.464.$$

The corresponding value for patients who are borderline positive is:

$$\frac{0.154}{0.154 + \dfrac{1 - 0.154}{0.2182 \div 0.1636}} = 0.195$$

and that for patients who have a negative result is:

$$\frac{0.154}{0.154 + \dfrac{1 - 0.154}{0.0909 \div 0.6909}} = 0.023$$

These values are the same (but for rounding) as those obtained in the series of all 357 patients where the predictive values could be calculated directly from the observed numbers (Table 2.7).

For a patient with a given result, the probability that he or she does *not* have an infarction is simply $1 - PV+$: "strong positives" $= 1 - 0.463 = 0.537$; "borderline positives" $= 1 - 0.196 = 0.804$; and "negatives" $= 1 - 0.023 = 0.977$, all numbers very close or equal to those seen in the table from the complete series of 357 patients (Table 2.7).

Single Measures of Test Validity

Some have given in to the temptation to summarize the assessment of the validity of a test with a single figure. Most commonly this is the percentage of patients correctly classified by the test. (This measure has been termed the "efficiency" of a test; see Galen and Gambino, 1975.) Using the myocardial infarction example shown in Table 2.1, the percentage would be:

$$\frac{(true\ positives) + (true\ negatives)}{total\ patients} \times 100 = \frac{50 + 211}{357} \times 100 = 73.1\%$$

Summary measures such as the "percent correctly classified"—even when applied to a test that simply provides a positive or negative result—should be avoided for at least 2 reasons. First, they do not fit into the decision-making process regarding the use of the test, as do the positive and negative predictive values. Second, they can give misleading results. For example, consider a test with a sensitivity of zero and a specificity of 100%, that is, a test that labels every subject as not having the condition. In the myocardial infarction example (Table 2.1), this completely valueless test would still correctly classify 84.6% of the subjects [(0 + 302) / 357 × 100], a value far higher than could be obtained using the clinical criteria (60.5%).

In Measuring a Test's Validity, with What Should the Test Result Be Compared?

The results of a test can be compared with a reference measure at the time of testing, such as the level of a physiologic parameter or the presence of a pathologic state, or also with the occurrence of an outcome at a later time.

For example, the blood pressure measured via a sphygmomanometer can be "validated" by simultaneous direct arterial measurement or by determining the extent to which it predicts the subsequent occurrence of morbid cardio-vascular events.

Under some circumstances, being able to determine the validity of a test result in assessing the physiologic or pathologic state can offer an excellent indication of the test's ability to predict the clinical outcome of concern. For example, consider a study that seeks to determine whether the results of fecal occult blood screening predict the *presence* of colorectal cancer. Even though the study is not assessing *mortality* from this disease, it offers a good idea of the ability of the test to predict who will and will not die from colorectal cancer: Persons who have colorectal cancer at a given point in time are at far higher risk than other persons of dying from it later on. In a similar way, because we believe hyperkalemia can cause cardiac arrest, a study of the accuracy of our laboratory test in measuring the true serum potassium level is, effectively, a study of the test's ability to predict cardiac arrest.

Nonetheless, in many instances it is desirable to have a direct assessment of the relation between the result of a test and the presence (or subsequent development) of the relevant clinical outcome(s). In this spirit, the investigation of Goldman et al. (1982) concerning the predictors of myocardial infarction in patients with chest pain was ultimately expanded to focus on predictors of untoward outcomes (i.e., *complications* of myocardial infarction) in these patients (Goldman et al., 1996). Among 10,682 persons with chest pain seen in the emergency departments of 7 hospitals, the researchers identified those who went on to develop a "major event" (e.g., cardiac arrest, cardiogenic shock, progression or recurrence of cardiac symptoms or signs that ultimately led to surgical intervention) during the first 12 hours. Based on EKG results, pain characteristics, and findings on physical examination, the investigators were able to identify 4 categories of patients whose likelihood of experiencing a "major event" ranged from 0.1% to 12.1%. Similar results were obtained when these same criteria were used to categorize a second set of 4,676 patients (Goldman et al., 1996). For a more complete appraisal of the data bearing on the possible stratification of patients with chest pain in terms of management strategies, see Lee and Goldman (2000).

Of course, no matter how accurate or how predictive a test, the test should not be performed unless its results either (a) enable interventions that lead, on average, to improved patient outcomes or (b) prevent the use of interventions that are not likely to improve outcome. Relevant patient outcomes include the incidence of a disease-related complication or the severity of those complications that do occur, as well as the incidence and/or severity of adverse effects of therapy. Approaches to measuring the extent to which the use of a test influences the occurrence of these outcomes are discussed next.

Questions

2.1. Three hundred men hospitalized for symptoms of urinary obstruction were evaluated for the presence of cancer of the prostate gland. Among the tests performed by their physicians (board-certified urologists) was a digital rectal examination. An examination was deemed positive if nodular irregularities or induration were present. This determination was made without knowledge of the results of other tests or of needle biopsy. The correspondence of the results of digital examination with those of biopsy is shown in the following table (Guinan et al., 1980):

Digital examination result	Biopsy positive for prostate cancer		
	Yes	No	Total
Positive	48	25	73
Negative	21	206	227
Total	69	231	300

We will assume that the biopsy results are completely accurate in assessing the presence or absence of prostate cancer.

a. In this population of men, what are the sensitivity and specificity of the digital examination for the presence of prostate cancer?

b. In this population of men, what is the predictive value of a positive result of a digital examination? A negative result?

c. You are a primary care physician considering administering an annual digital rectal examination to men in your practice over 50 years of age who have no symptoms of prostate cancer. From reviewing the literature, you suspect the prevalence of prostate cancer in this group to be about 0.5%. (i) Using the sensitivity and specificity obtained in 2.1a for the men with urological symptoms, calculate the fraction of men with a positive digital examination result who should prove to have prostate cancer. (ii) This proportion (predictive value of a positive test) is lower than the one calculated in 2.1b. Why? (iii) What reservations do you have in applying the values for sensitivity and specificity of the digital examination obtained for the urological patients to values that might be found in your practice?

2.2. The following is excerpted from an article on the early detection of endometrial cancer.

From a screening pool of approximately 300,000 Papanicolaou tests, 177 women had cervical cytologic studies, involving an exocervical scrape and endocervical swab, that demonstrated atypical endometrial

cells. Of these 177 women, 134 underwent additional diagnostic procedures within 12 months of their cytologic evaluation. Adenocarcinoma
of the endometrium was observed in 27 (20%) of the 134 women with
atypical endometrial cells.

In assessing the validity of the finding of atypical endometrial cells in
detecting carcinoma of the endometrium, which of the following measures
can be estimated from the data provided here: (a) sensitivity, (b) specificity,
(c) predictive value of a positive test, (d) predictive value of a negative test?
For those measures that can be estimated, what are the estimates? For those
that cannot be estimated, what additional data are needed?

2.3. You are an obstetrician interested in determining whether the presence
of oligohydramnios (reduced volume of amniotic fluid) detectable on ultrasound screening early in pregnancy is predictive of a spontaneous abortion in
that pregnancy. Over a period of several years, you and your colleagues have
identified 32 pregnant women in whom oligohydramnios was present. Thirty
went on to have spontaneous abortions. For purposes of comparison, from 3
scattered weeks during this time period you identify 52 women who received
the same screening test but were found not to have oligohydramnios. Only
4 of them had subsequent spontaneous abortions. In assessing the degree
to which the presence of oligohydramnios (detectable via early ultrasound
screening) predicts spontaneous abortion, which of the following measures
can be estimated from the data provided here: (a) sensitivity (of the presence
of oligohydramnios in predicting spontaneous abortion), (b) specificity, (c)
predictive value of a positive test, (d) predictive value of a negative test? For
those measures that can be estimated, what are the estimates?

2.4. Accurate prediction of fetal lung maturity can aid in the management
of pregnancy in several ways, for example, in the timing of elective cesarean
section to minimize the risk of respiratory distress syndrome (RDS) in the
newborn infant. Fluorescence polarization (FP), a measure of the relative
amount of surfactant in amniotic fluid, appears to provide a relatively accurate prediction in most cases. For example, in one study (Chen et al., 1992)
of consecutive samples of amniotic fluid sent for FP analysis, 53 of 77 infants
who later developed RDS had FP values of > 0.29 polarization units, in contrast to only 24 of 471 infants who did not develop RDS. Only 5 of the 787
cases had FP values < 0.26, in contrast to 394 of the 471 normal infants.

In the "intermediate" range of values for the FP test—0.260 to 0.289 polarization units—there were 19 RDS cases and 53 normal infants, and a result in
this range was not felt to offer much clinical guidance. A group of investigators wanted to determine whether another test, the ratio of lecithin/sphingo-
myelin (L/S) in amniotic fluid, might help to discriminate RDS cases from
noncases when the FP result fell into this intermediate range. The L/S test
had been performed on 55 of these 72 samples, including 17/19 (89.5%) of

the RDS cases and 38/53 (71.7%) of the normal infants whose FP values had been intermediate. The following results were obtained:

L/S in amniotic fluid[a]	RDS	No RDS
< 2.0	10	17
> 2.0	7	21

[a] In specimens in which the FP result was 0.260–0.289 polarization units.

Among amniotic fluid specimens that gave an "intermediate" FP result (i.e., 0.260–0.289), what is the predictive value for RDS of a "positive" L/S test (i.e., <2.0)? What is the predictive value of a "negative" L/S test (i.e., >2.0)? How do these predictive values compare with the probability of RDS given an FP result of 0.260–0.289 if no L/S result had been available?

2.5. The following is paraphrased from an article on screening for ovarian cancer:

The incidence of ovarian cancer in European and North American women aged 45 years or over is about 1 in 2,500 per year. Therefore, a screening test for ovarian cancer, even with 100% sensitivity, would require 99.6% specificity to achieve a positive predictive value of 10% (i.e., 9 false positive tests for each case of ovarian cancer identified). Because even a small fall in specificity would produce a large decrease in the predictive value, and because the consequence of a positive screening test often is surgical intervention, high specificity is an essential requirement of any screening test for ovarian cancer.

a. Show how the authors determined that, given a test with 100% sensitivity, a specificity of 99.6% would be needed to achieve a positive predictive value of 10%.

b. Instead of the annual incidence of ovarian cancer, what is the appropriate measure the authors should have employed in calculating the needed specificity of a test? Why is it preferable to annual incidence?

Answers

2.1.a. Sensitivity = 48/69 = 69.6%
      Specificity = 206/231 = 89.2%
  b. $PV+$ = 48/73 = 65.8%
      $PV-$ = 206/227 = 90.7%
  c(i). In a population of 10,000 men in which 50 have prostate cancer:

| | Prostate cancer | | |
Digital examination	Yes	No	Total[a]
Positive	a	b	
Negative	c	d	
Total[a]	50	9,950	10,000

[a] This number is arbitrary

$a = 50(48/69) = 35$

$c = 50 - a = 15$

$d = 9,950(206/231) = 8,873$

$b = 9,950 - d = 1,077$

| | Prostate cancer | | |
Digital examination	Yes	No	Total
Positive	35	1,077	1,112
Negative	15	8,873	8,888
Total	50	9,950	10,000

$$PV+ = 35/1,112 \times 100 = 3.1\%$$

c(ii). Only 3.1% of your screened patients who have a positive digital exam will turn out to have prostate cancer. This $PV+$ is lower than that obtained for the men with urological symptoms because the prevalence of prostate cancer differs so much between the groups: 0.5% in the asymptomatic men versus 23% (69/300) in those with urological symptoms.

c(iii). Because most of the patients you are examining will not have urological symptoms, the average size of any tumors that are present will probably be smaller than that found in a series of symptomatic men. Thus the ability of the digital examination to detect true positives in this group may be lower (i.e., lower sensitivity). Also, the sensitivity of the examination may be related to the skill of the person performing it; quite possibly the urologists are more adept at this examination than you are. Those 2 factors, which could act to decrease the sensitivity of digital examination in your patients relative to that found in the published study, would also lower the $PV+$.

In addition, the specificity of the digital examination obtained in the study of patients with urological symptoms also may not predict that which you would achieve in your practice. Again, your relative lack of expertise may lead to a greater proportion of false positives (i.e., lower specificity). On the other hand, among your screened patients who do not have prostate cancer, the large majority will not have other prostate abnormalities that could mimic cancer on the digital examination. Thus your proportion of false positives could actually be smaller, leading to a higher $PV+$ than that estimated in c(i).

The moral of the story: Results of diagnostic tests performed by others, on patient populations other than the one you are dealing with, can only be a guide to how well the test will perform for you. How good a guide they will be is a function of the variability of the test when performed by different individuals (laboratories, radiology departments, etc.), as well as of the similarity of the populations being tested.

2.2. From the data provided, the following table can be constructed:

Atypical endometrial cells	Adenocarcinoma of the endometrium		
	Yes	No	Total
Yes	27	107	134
No	?	?	
	?	?	

The predictive value of a positive test is $27/134 \times 100 = 20.1\%$. None of the other 3 measures of test accuracy can be calculated. In order to do so, data would have to be obtained on the prevalence of endometrial cancer among women whose tests did *not* reveal atypical endometrial cells.

2.3. Of 32 women with oligohydramnios, all but 2 subsequently experienced spontaneous abortion: the positive predictive value is $30/32 = 93.8\%$. The predictive value of an ultrasound exam that is negative for oligohydramnios is $48/52 = 92.3\%$. Because of the way in which subjects were chosen for the study (all women detected as having oligohydramnios, but only a small sample of other women), it is not possible to estimate from these data alone the sensitivity and specificity of the test result. Valid estimates of these measures can be obtained only if: (a) the proportion of women with and without ultrasound-detectable oligohydramnios in the sample reflects the proportion present in the underlying population of pregnant women seeking care from the obstetricians or (b) that proportion in the underlying population is known.

Oligohydramnios	Spontaneous abortion		
	Yes	No	Total
Yes	30	2	32
No	4	48	52

2.4. Among infants with an amniotic fluid FP value of 0.260–0.289, the probability of RDS is

$$\frac{19}{19 + 53} + 26.4\%,$$

not

$$\frac{17}{17 + 38} + 30.9\%,$$

This must be taken into account when estimating the $PV+$ and $PV-$ of the L/S test.

$$PV+ = \frac{.264(10/17)}{.264(10/17) + .736(17/38)} = 32.0\%,$$

versus a risk of RDS of 26.4% if no L/S result had been available.

$$PV- = \frac{.736(21/38)}{.736(21/38) + .264(7/17)} = 78.9\%,$$

versus a likelihood of no RDS of 73.6% if no L/S result had been available.

2.5.a. In a population of 250,000 women (this number is arbitrary), a universally applied screening test for a disease present in 100 of the women that had (a) a sensitivity of 100% and (b) a positive predictive value of 10% would categorize the women as follows:

	Ovarian cancer		
Test result	Present	Absent	Total
Positive	100	900	1000
Negative	0	d	d
Total	100	249,900	250,000

By subtraction, the number of women without ovarian cancer who test as negative ("d") is 249,000. The specificity of such a test must then be

$$\frac{249,000}{249,900} \times 100\% = 99.6\%,$$

b. The test is seeking to identify women who have an otherwise occult ovarian cancer that is nonetheless sufficiently advanced to be detectable. Therefore, instead of the incidence of clinically evident ovarian cancer, what is needed to estimate the required specificity of the test is the prevalence of occult but potentially detectable ovarian cancer.

References

Begg CB. Biases in the assessment of diagnostic tests. *Stat Med* 1987;6:411–423.

Chen C, Roby PV, Weiss NS, et al. Clinical evaluation of the NBD-PC fluorescence polarization assay for prediction of fetal lung maturity. *Obstet Gynecol* 1992;80:688–692.

Freedman LS. Statistical methods of evaluating and comparing imaging techniques. In Bleehen NM, ed. *Investigational Techniques in Oncology.* London: Springer-Verlag; 1987.

Galen RD, Gambino SR. *Beyond Normality: The Predictive Value and Efficiency of Medical Diagnosis.* New York: John Wiley; 1975.

Goldman L, Weinberg M, Weisberg M, et al. A computer-derived protocol to aid in the diagnosis of emergency room patients with acute chest pain. *N Engl J Med* 1982;307:588–596.

Goldman L, Cook EF, Johnson PA, et al. Prediction of the need for intensive care in patients who come to emergency departments with chest pain. *N Engl J Med* 1996;334:1498–1504.

Guinan P, Bush I, Ray V, et al. The accuracy of the rectal examination in the diagnosis of prostate carcinoma. *N Engl J Med* 1980;303:499–503.

Lee TH, Goldman L. Evaluation of the patient with acute chest pain. *N Engl J Med* 2000;342:1187–1194.

Wasson JH, Sox HC, Neff RK, et al. Clinical prediction rules: Applications and methodological standards. *N Engl J Med* 1985;313:793–799.

3

Diagnostic and Screening Tests

Measuring Their Role in Improving the Outcome of Illness

Ordering or performing a diagnostic or screening test can reduce the frequency of disease occurrence (or progression, or complications) only if the test can (a) detect the condition or abnormality before it or its consequences would otherwise be evident, and (b) lead to treatment that is more effective when administered soon after the time of testing than if it were to be administered either later in the natural history of the condition, when the condition or abnormality becomes evident in the absence of testing, or not administered at all.

To introduce the alternative ways by which we can assess the benefit a test can produce, let's consider 2 groups of 10,000 middle-aged and elderly adults. In one of the groups, screening for high blood pressure takes place, but otherwise the groups are identical. For simplicity, assume that the screening leads to the identification of just 2 categories of patients in terms of subsequent treatment recommendations: hypertensives and normotensives. In the group not screened, the all-cause mortality after 5 years would be a function of that in hypertensive and normotensive persons, although, of course, neither would have been identified as such:

Table 3.1. All-Cause Mortality in a Population in Which There Was No Screening for High Blood Pressure

Blood pressure	Death within 5 years		
	Yes	No	Total
Hypertensive	90	810	900
Normotensive	455	8,645	9,100
Total	545	9,455	10,000

Assume that in the screened group the 900 hypertensive persons were accurately identified (sensitivity and specificity = 100%) and treated, and that their mortality was but 70% that of untreated hypertensives. The mortality experience of this group of 10,000 persons would be as follows:

Table 3.2.   All-Cause Mortality in a Population in Which
Screening for High Blood Pressure Has Taken Place

Blood pressure	Death within 5 years		
	Yes	No	Total
Hypertensive	$90 \times 0.7 = 63$	837	900
Normotensive	455	8,645	9,100
Total	518	9,482	10,000

The reduction in the population's mortality achieved by blood pressure screening would be 27 deaths per 10,000. This represents only a (545 − 518)/545 = 5% difference from the population's mortality rate in the absence of screening. To convincingly demonstrate (in a statistical sense) a difference of this magnitude, a study would have to be *very* large—approximately 100,000 screened and 100,000 unscreened subjects would be needed. These large numbers arise in part because the mortality follow-up cannot be confined to persons with high blood pressure—the only group capable of being benefited. Because in the unscreened population no person's blood pressure would be known to the investigator, the occurrence of death in all persons in this population needs to be monitored. For purposes of comparability, deaths in all members of the screened population, hypertensives and normotensives, would need to be monitored as well.

Fortunately, the degree to which the use of a test leads to improved patient outcomes often can be estimated through a more feasible approach than a direct comparison of the rate with which those outcomes occur in large numbers of persons who do and do not receive that test. This approach involves obtaining 3 separate pieces of information:

1. The proportion of the tested population with a positive test result;
2. The ability of the test result to detect the condition or abnormality before it or its consequences would otherwise be evident; and
3. The effectiveness of treatment among test-positive persons.

In the example of screening for blood pressure, let's say we locate the relevant information for persons whom we suspect to be similar to those we are considering as candidates for testing. It indicates that:

1. Nine percent of screened patients are hypertensive;
2. After 5 years, 10% of persons found to have high blood pressure have died, in contrast to 5% of normotensive individuals; and

    3. Treated hypertensives have 70% the mortality of untreated hyper-
       tensives.

Armed with this information, we can readily produce data for 2 hypothetical populations, one tested, the other not, that are identical to the data
found in Tables 3.1 and 3.2. In a group of 10,000 unscreened persons, 900
(9%) would have hypertension, of whom 90 (10%) would die, during the
ensuing 5 years. Of the 9,100 normotensives, 455 (5%) would die, for a total
mortality of 545 per 10,000. In 10,000 screened persons, now that those with
hypertension have been identified and treated, there would be 63 (70% of
90) hypertensives who would be predicted to have died. The 5-year mortality
among normotensive persons would not have changed, so there would be a
total of 518 deaths (63 + 455).

From the foregoing example, it is clear that the information that allows
us to piece together tables such as 3.1 and 3.2 can be generated in separate
studies. Our knowledge of the rate of illness or complications conditional
on a test result (number 2 in the preceding list) generally will arise from a
study devoted specifically to this issue. Studies of this type are discussed
in Chapter 7. Sometimes, however, the illness or complication rates in test-
positive persons can be gleaned from the experience of untreated (or placebo-
treated) patients in a randomized trial that has been done primarily to assess
therapeutic efficacy (number 3 in the preceding list; see Chapter 4).

The measurement of the frequency with which positive tests occur among
patients with a given indication for testing (number 1 in the preceding list)
often requires an entirely separate study. For example, among several series of infants and toddlers with unexplained fevers, investigators systematically have obtained blood cultures to determine the frequency of occult
bacteremia (Teele et al., 1975; Schwartz and Wientzen, 1982; Kramer et al.,
1986). As another example, several pediatricians sought to evaluate the utility of follow-up chest X-rays in children diagnosed as having pneumonia
3–4 weeks earlier but who no longer had any symptoms or signs (Gibson et
al., 1993). Of 59 such children identified by investigators, none had X-ray
evidence of effusion, persisting collapse, or any other abnormality that had
a bearing on further treatment. Although the prevalence of abnormal X-rays
in *all* children with this particular indication for being tested is certainly
not zero (see Hanley and Lippman-Hand, 1983, for estimating the maximum
frequency of positive tests compatible with the observed findings), studies
of this type give guidance as to the maximal impact a test could be expected
to have in a given clinical setting.

The evidence in support of the efficacy of the large majority of tests currently in use comes from aggregating the results of studies that evaluate
one (or at most two) of the component questions that need to be addressed.
Screening for high blood pressure is believed to be efficacious because separate studies have shown high blood pressure to be a common characteristic,
one that can predispose to premature mortality to a substantial degree but

that does so to a considerably lesser extent if it is treated. Similarly, we have a good idea of the benefit that regular retinal examination can have in preventing blindness in diabetics, because we know:

1. The prevalence of retinopathy in diabetics;
2. That retinal examination by trained practitioners can identify diabetic retinopathy with high sensitivity and specificity (Moss et al., 1985) and that retinopathy so identified is an extremely strong predictor of blindness; and
3. That laser photocoagulation therapy for retinopathy can reduce the occurrence of severe visual impairment (Early Treatment Diabetic Retinopathy Study Group, 1987).

But what is to be done if all patients who are found to be "positive" on a certain test happen to receive treatment? Persons who are tested for the presence of cancer and found to have it, for example, are almost never left untreated. Thus, although it is not difficult to determine that a number of screening tests for cancer can detect the disease earlier than it would be detected otherwise (e.g., by comparing the distribution of tumor size or stage in screened and unscreened persons with that cancer), it is usually not possible to answer the next necessary question: Does treatment given at the time of early detection lead to a more favorable outcome than treatment given when the cancer is clinically manifest? In situations such as this, it is necessary to resort to the more cumbersome design referred to earlier: a comparison of the subsequent occurrence of progression of complications in tested and untested persons. This design is assessing jointly the frequency of test positivity, the ability of the test result to predict an adverse outcome, and the efficacy of treatment for test-positive individuals, and it will hereafter be referred to as a "one-step" design.

The remainder of this chapter outlines the types of one-step designs available to evaluate a test's ability to lead to improved patient outcomes.

Randomized Trials and Cohort (Follow-Up) Studies

The study participants can be assigned at random to receive or not receive the test (or a program of testing). Alternatively, it is possible to exploit (with appropriate caution when interpreting the results) the fact that in the normal course of medical or public health practice, some persons are tested whereas others are not, and these 2 groups can be monitored for the outcome(s) of interest.

An example of the first type of one-step design is the randomized trial conducted in England on the efficacy of ultrasound screening for abdominal aortic aneurysms (Multicentre Aneurysm Screening Study Group, 2002). During 1997–1999, 33,839 men from 4 parts of the country were randomly selected from family doctor and Health Authority lists to be invited to attend a screening exam, and 80% accepted the invitation. Another 33,961 men identified on these lists served as controls. Men found to have an aneurysm ≥ 3 cm in diameter who did not meet specific criteria (based primarily on size and symptoms) for prompt surgery underwent periodic repeat ultrasound exams. Deaths were identified through the Office of National Statistics mortality surveillance system. Those deaths characterized by a review panel (blinded as to the screening status of individual study participants) as being aneurysm related were more numerous in the control group (113; 3.3 per 1,000 men) than in men invited for screening (65; 1.9 per 1,000 men) ($p = 0.0002$) during the 4-year follow-up period.

Randomized trials have now been conducted to evaluate the efficacy of a variety of diagnostic and screening tests, including, as examples, prenatal ultrasound exams (Ewigman et al., 1993; Bucher and Schmidt, 1993), intrapartum fetal heart rate monitoring (Mahomed et al., 1994), routine cervical evaluation during pregnancy (Buekens et al., 1994), electronic home uterine monitoring in women at high risk of premature delivery (U.S. Preventive Services Task Force, 1993), mammography and clinical breast exam (Shapiro et al., 1982), breast self-examination (Thomas et al., 2002), and fecal occult blood screening (Mandel et al., 1993).

Some randomized trials contrast the outcomes that occur among patients assigned to receive one of two tests for a given indication. These trials have no untested group and so are suitable only when there is already evidence that one of the tests leads, on average, to an improved outcome. For example, Dronfield et al. (1977) randomized patients hospitalized for acute upper gastrointestinal tract bleeding to receive an endoscopic or radiologic evaluation. Though endoscopy produced a higher likelihood of identifying a lesion responsible for the blood loss (108/162 = 67%) than did radiology (88/160 = 55%), there were no appreciable differences between the groups regarding the occurrence of surgery or death during that hospitalization.

The second type of one-step assessment of a test's ability to influence the outcome of illness is exemplified by the comparison of neonatal mortality among children delivered by mothers who received fetal monitoring during labor with that among children whose mothers had not been monitored (Neutra et al., 1978). This nonrandomized follow-up study took place in a hospital during a period of time in which fetal monitoring was being introduced. The choice of patients to undergo monitoring was made by each woman's physician, not by the investigators (who conducted the study in retrospect through the use of the hospital's records).

Ideally, all evaluations of diagnostic or screening test efficacy would be randomized: Assignment of patients to test or no-test groups in a random way assures that the only differences between the two groups that might be relevant to the outcome in question are those that occur by chance. This is decidedly not the case in nonrandomized studies, as there may be important differences that can distort (i.e., confound) the true benefit, or lack thereof, associated with use of the test. In the fetal monitoring study, for example, the investigators discovered in their review of records that a relatively higher proportion of mothers who did not receive monitoring had characteristics that predict an increased risk of mortality in the child: short gestation, breech presentation, placenta previa, and so on. Failure to have taken into account these differences in the analysis would have resulted in a comparison erroneously favorable to the monitored group and would have led to an overestimation of the benefit associated with monitoring.

Unfortunately, even when it is possible in the course of a nonrandomized study to measure and to take into account the influence of some confounding variables, it is never possible to be sure that there are not others. For example, there may have been characteristics other than short gestation or breech presentation associated with not administering fetal monitoring to women that also had a strong bearing on neonatal mortality. The likelihood with which unmeasured factors are biasing (confounding) the results often can be guessed at, as can the degree to which they may be doing so. For this reason, the results of nonrandomized studies, particularly those suggesting a substantial degree of efficacy, are commonly used in arriving at decisions regarding the use of diagnostic and screening tests. Nonetheless, these results are never as "satisfying" as would be the same results from an otherwise comparable randomized study. (Also see Chapter 5 for a more complete discussion of the strengths and limitations of nonrandomized evaluations.)

There are some nonrandomized follow-up studies in which the potential for bias due to confounding is particularly clear. Perhaps you are attempting to evaluate the success of a blood lead screening program for preschool children in which the test was available to all who requested it. The program's "success" would be measured by IQ testing of these children once they were of school age, and their performance would be compared with that of an unscreened group. Not having been able to assign children at random to the test or no-test categories, you are fearful that the two groups of children may have IQ differences based on a number of other factors (e.g., parental IQ differences) apart from any benefit the screening program may have had. It may even be that the screened children had some neurological or behavioral problems that were the reason for their being tested. If it is not possible to identify these other factors and measure them comparably in screened and unscreened children, the results of any comparison will have little credibility.

A number of nonrandomized evaluations of the efficacy of screening for cancer provide additional examples of these same problems. Records available to the study may not be adequate to determine: (a) the degree to which tested and untested persons differ in terms of their underlying risks of the cancer toward which the test is targeted; and (b) whether among tested individuals, symptoms or signs of that cancer were present that stimulated them to seek testing (Weiss et al., 2004).

Which Subjects Are to Be Compared?

In most evaluations of the efficacy of diagnostic or screening tests, the only comparison that can be made is of the overall occurrence of progression or complications in the screened versus unscreened groups. In a blood lead screening evaluation, for instance, one would compare the prevalence of retardation in children who did and did not receive screening. The lead levels in the unscreened group would never be known, so even if the investigators wished to compare outcomes in only those persons with elevated levels in each group, it would be impossible to do so.

Some conditions for which testing is done will, after a period of time, be evident even without the benefit of the test. Most cancers fall into this category, and there has been a temptation to evaluate the efficacy of cancer screening tests by comparing mortality from the particular cancer in cases found through screening with that in other cases. Giving in to this temptation will lead to erroneous results, primarily due to the influence of what is known as lead-time bias.

The reason for this bias is illustrated in the following example. Suppose 100 individuals are screened for cancer X, a cancer for which there is no effective treatment. On the average, the test succeeds in identifying the cancer 1 year before it is clinically evident. Four persons in the group are detected as having cancer X, and the course of their illness is shown in Figure 3.1.

Two deaths occur among the 4 persons with cancer X in the 13 person-years following screening (3 + 4 + 2 + 4; see Figure 3.1), and the mortality rate in this group is 2 per 13 person-years. Had the screening *not* been performed, however, the same 2 deaths among 4 cases in 100 persons would occur (because no effective treatment follows early detection).

But the number of person-years accruing in these cases from the time of their diagnosis (1 year later than that for the screened cases) would be only 9 (2 + 3 + 1 + 3), and the resulting mortality rate would be higher, 2 per 9 person-years. Because screening could not lead to improved mortality, one must conclude that there is something faulty in this method of comparison. (If, instead of using mortality rates, the measure of outcome were n-year survival, the bias would still be present. Thus the 1.5-year survival in the cases found through screening is 100%, whereas the 1.5-year survival in the other cases is 75%, even though the two groups had, in truth, an identical survival experience.)

What is faulty, of course, is that the starting point for monitoring mortality rates is different between the screened and unscreened cases, always to the apparent detriment of the cases detected without screening. The appropriate comparison to make is the mortality experience (with respect to that cancer) not of the cases alone but of the screened group with that of an unscreened group, *with both groups monitored from the time of screening.* In the preceding example, the mortality rate in the screened group is 2 deaths in 397 person-years (98 persons × 4 years, plus 1 person × 2 years, plus 1 person

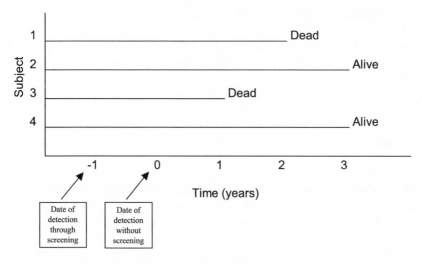

Figure 3.1 Lead time in studies of the efficacy of screening.

× 3 years). In a comparable unscreened group, the rate would be the same, because the number of person-years, counted from the time the screening would have taken place had it been done, is identical to that for the screened group. Given that the natural history of this cancer is not altered by screening, this comparison of screened and unscreened groups, which indicates no benefit associated with screening, is clearly the preferred one.

Patients who have a long preclinical-but-detectable phase of disease are more readily found via screening than are patients with that disease whose preclinical phase is short. To the extent that the length of the preclinical phase correlates with the length of the illness once it has been detected, those persons whose disease was found via screening will appear to have a better survival rate, even in the absence of treatment that influences the disease's natural history. This possible artifact, due to what has been termed "length-biased sampling" (Zelen, 1976), is another reason that a comparison of survival in persons whose disease was detected by screening with that of other diseased persons will be misleading.

Other Nonrandomized Approaches to Measuring the Degree to Which Tests Reduce the Occurrence of Disease Progression or Complications

Population Comparisons

Let's say you are interested in determining whether the routine hospitalization of persons with acute chest pain reduces mortality from myocardial infarction in comparison with a policy of hospitalizing only those patients who meet certain clinical criteria based on EKG abnormalities and the characteristics of their chest pain. You despair of obtaining the resources necessary to identify and follow the large number of persons needed for a nonrandomized follow-up study, and a randomized trial seems even less feasible. What about simply comparing the mortality rates from acute myocardial infarction in two or more populations whose experience differs regarding routine hospitalization? The "populations" could be defined, for example, according to residence in certain geographic areas in which care was provided. Data would have to be available on the occurrence of the complication (e.g., death from myocardial infarction) and, at least roughly, on the degree to which one or the other of the testing strategies (i.e., selective vs. routine admission) had been employed in the respective populations. What is not needed for this type of comparison is the more difficult to come by knowledge of both test and complication status in individual patients—if these were known, a nonrandomized follow-up design could be used.

Although population comparisons offer a relatively inexpensive and rapid means of assessing test efficacy, it is only under unusual circumstances that the evidence they provide can be considered anything more than suggestive. The reason is that it is uncommon to find populations that differ to a large degree in the use they make of a diagnostic or screening test but that are otherwise similar with respect to (a) the rate of occurrence of the outcome that can result from progression or complications of the condition for which testing is being done and (b) the completeness and accuracy of the reporting of this outcome.

Occurrence of the Condition

One way to evaluate the efficacy of a blood lead screening program in reducing the prevalence of mental retardation is to compare the prevalence of the retardation in the screened population, after the screening has been initiated, with that of one or more unscreened populations. The latter would be chosen on the basis of characteristics that would predict a frequency of retardation identical to that of the screened population save for the influence of screening. Such characteristics might be geographic proximity to the screened population, income level, age and type of housing, and the use of similar methods of identifying retarded children.

The difficulty in interpreting the results of such a comparison is that, despite our best efforts in selecting control communities, we are never very sure that the "background" prevalences of retardation among the populations were indeed similar. Might the difference (or lack thereof) we observe in the prevalence of retardation have been present in the absence of screening? This is particularly a problem if the screening measure, by its nature, is unlikely to have a dramatic impact on the overall occurrence of the complication or condition it seeks to prevent. For instance, because lead exposure may be responsible for only a relatively small fraction of the retardation that occurs among children, even an effective screening program may make only a small dent in the overall prevalence, which would be hard to detect against the background level.

Completeness and Accuracy of Reporting

Often it is difficult to obtain comparable data across populations on the occurrence of the adverse outcome of interest, particularly in a population group large enough to provide enough instances of progression or complications for a meaningful contrast. For example, a comparison of routinely available mortality rates for myocardial infarction between two cities or states probably would not be a sensitive measure of the impact of any differences between them that stem from different policies for hospitalization of persons with acute chest pain—such rates easily could be differentially inaccurate between the populations.

Occasionally, the circumstances under which population comparisons are made allow results to be interpreted with relatively great confidence.

Example: A program of cervical screening of Icelandic women aged 25 to 59 years was begun in 1964. Whereas only occasionally would women have received screening prior to that time, by the early 1970s some 80% of the target population had been examined at the screening clinic. Some women 60 years of age and over were screened as well, but not in any appreciable numbers until after 1970. The mortality from cervical cancer and the incidence of lesions diagnosed at Stage II or greater are shown in Table 3.3. In 25- to 59-year-old women, a rise both in mortality and in the incidence of late-stage disease during 1955 through 1969 was reversed in the years 1970–1974. In women 60 to 89 years old, the group that underwent little screening, there was no systematic variation in either rate during the interval (Johannesson et al., 1978).

Table 3.3.   Cervical Cancer in Iceland, 1955 to 1974

Age (years)	Measure	Rate of cervical cancer[a]			
		1955–1959	1960–1964	1965–1969	1970–1974
25–59	Mortality	11.7	16.8	26.5	12.2
	Incidence, Stage II +	16.8	19.3	22.3	11.8
60–89	Mortality	27.6	33.3	28.2	34.8
	Incidence, Stage II +	27.8	21.0	25.4	23.1

[a] Annual rate per 100,000, age-adjusted (5-year groups) to a uniform standard.
Source: Johannesson et al. (1978)

Was it the screening that was responsible for this difference between the "populations" (i.e., the 25- to 59-year-old Icelandic women before and after the mass screening)? Features of the study's design and results that favor an affirmative answer to this question are as follows:

1. The difference in the level of screening between the time periods was very great, rising from near zero before 1964 to 80% within 10 years.
2. Reliable data were available on the mortality from cervical cancer.
3. The size of the population in each time period was sufficiently large to provide enough cervical cancer deaths for meaningful analysis.
4. There is evidence to indicate that in the absence of screening, the mortality rates among 25- to 59-year-old women would not have fallen: (a) Prior to the introduction of mass screening, the rates in women in this age group actually had been on the increase; and (b) in those Icelandic women who were largely unscreened, that is, women aged 60 to 89, there was no corresponding decrease in mortality from cervical cancer during 1970 through 1974.
5. The mortality (and late-stage incidence) in the years 1970–1974 was reduced to such a large degree that it is implausible that other, un-measured changes during the period could have been solely respon-sible.

These are precisely the features that are rarely present together in most comparisons of populations.

Case-Control Studies

The case-control approach is particularly valuable when studying disease etiology, and it plays an important role in evaluating therapeutic safety (see Chapter 6). It examines potential associations between exposures and disease in what at first seems an illogical way, that is, by comparing the frequency (or level) of exposure in a group of persons having a disease with that in an otherwise comparable group of persons without it. Although the opportunity for bias in such studies is considerable (as is the case for any nonrandomized study), if properly done they have the potential to provide an accurate esti-mate of the relative disease incidence in exposed and nonexposed persons (Cornfield, 1951) and can do so in an efficient way.

How can this type of study design be put to use to evaluate the efficacy of a diagnostic or screening test? "Cases" would have to be defined as in-dividuals who have developed progressive disease or those complications that one is seeking to prevent by prompt diagnosis. "Controls" would be de-fined as persons without progression or complications but who are otherwise comparable. Thus, if the cases were persons who died of colorectal cancer, controls would be selected so as to be representative of the population at risk for development of colorectal cancer at the time the cases were diagnosed. Records of the 2 groups would be examined to determine which persons had undergone screening (for the presence of fecal occult blood, for example) during a period of time prior to diagnosis in which a tumor plausibly could be identified by the test (or, for controls, a corresponding period). The data would be displayed as follows:

Screening for fecal occult blood	Death from colorectal cancer	
	Yes	No
Performed	a	b
Not performed	c	d

In asymptomatic persons, testing for fecal occult blood would be effective in reducing mortality in proportion to the amount by which $b/(b + d)$ exceeded $a/(a + c)$ (Weiss et al., 1992). The relative mortality from colorectal cancer associated with a history of screening during this interval would equal the relative odds of screening between cases and controls, that is,

$$(a/c) / (b/d).$$

(See Chapter 6 for the derivation of this formula.) If, perhaps, 20% of persons who died of colorectal cancer had undergone screening for fecal occult blood during the 2-year period ending just before diagnosis, in contrast to 30% of controls during the same interval, the relative mortality associated with screening would be

$$(20/80) / (30/70) = 0.58.$$

The use of the case-control study to measure the efficacy of *diagnostic* tests has, to the present time, been more a theoretical possibility than a reality. The reason is that the conditions required for such studies have rarely been present: (a) a large patient population for which data regarding symptoms are uniformly available and (b) a patient population within which there is variation in the frequency (or speed) with which diagnostic tests are used.

Case-control studies of the efficacy of *screening* tests have proven somewhat more feasible, primarily because there is often more variability in the occurrence of screening in healthy persons than in the use of diagnostic tests in sick ones. Three features of the design and analysis of case-control studies of screening efficacy are worthy of mention.

1. Persons selected as cases should be ill or disabled to a degree that diagnosis would occur in the absence of screening (Morrison, 1982). For a disease such as cancer, the criterion for selection could be death from cancer (or possibly the presence of late-stage disease that is not believed to be curable), irrespective of the stage at which the cancer was first diagnosed. In choosing cases for a study of blood lead screening and mental retardation, particular

care would have to be taken to set criteria stringent enough so that, in the study locale, cases of defined severity would be reliably identified even if no screening program existed.

2. Persons selected as controls should be representative of the population that generated the cases with respect to the presence and/or level of screening activity (Weiss, 1983). A control group restricted to persons with earlier or less severe forms of the condition under study (e.g., early-stage cancer) is not appropriate. The fact that the condition is detected early in such persons is probably the result of their having been screened. Thus, even if screening were not followed by any effective therapy, a case-control difference would exist: The controls' level of screening would be higher than that of the population from which the cases arose, falsely suggesting a benefit associated with screening. A bias of this sort is the case-control analogue of lead-time bias in follow-up studies. Although the appropriate control group would not exclude persons with early or mild disease, it would include them only in proportion to their numbers in the population. (What specifically constitutes an "appropriate" control group in a case-control study is a question that is discussed more fully in Chapter 6.)

Thus, in a case-control study that seeks to determine whether cytologic screening for cervical cancer leads to a reduction in mortality from the disease, one would not choose as controls women with in situ lesions. The presence of in situ cervical neoplasia is rarely discovered in the absence of screening, and so virtually every member of the control group will have had at least one screening examination. It is unlikely that such a high level of screening activity would occur among women in the population that gave rise to the patients who died from cervical cancer. The selection of women with in situ cancer as controls would produce a finding of apparent benefit from cytologic screening even if there were no effective treatment for the lesions discovered in this way.

> *Example:* Several case-control studies have been conducted to estimate the degree to which mortality from breast cancer might be reduced by early detection through regular breast self-examination (BSE). In some studies, women whose cancers were diagnosed at late and early stages (i.e., cases and controls, respectively) were compared with respect to the frequency of BSE. This design violates both principles thus far enumerated:
>
> (1) The goal of early detection is to prevent the occurrence of late-stage disease at any time, not merely at diagnosis. Thus the criteria for selection of "cases" should not have been based solely on information available at the time of diagnosis. Many cases who should have appeared (but did not) in these studies—women who developed late-stage breast cancer only at some time after the initial diagnosis of their disease—may have had early cancer found by BSE. Failure to include them in the case group would falsely inflate the measured efficacy of BSE.

(2) The BSE practices of women with breast cancer diagnoses at an early stage are almost certainly not typical of those of the population of women from which the late-stage cases arose. In most instances, BSE or other early-detection activity will have been responsible for the early diagnosis. Restriction of the control group to these women with higher than average early-detection activity will cause the control-case difference in the frequency of BSE to be falsely large and thus the estimate of relative mortality from breast cancer in women who perform BSE to be falsely low.

Case-control studies that seek to estimate the degree of reduction in breast cancer mortality afforded by BSE need to choose, as cases, women who develop metastatic breast cancer (i.e., women who are very likely to die of the disease) during a defined period of time, irrespective of the date of diagnosis of their primary tumor. As controls, such studies should identify a representative sample of women at risk for the development of breast cancer in that population from which the cases arose.

3. As is the case with all nonrandomized strategies for assessing the efficacy of screening, there is a possibility of obtaining a spurious result unless factors that are correlated both with the level of screening activity and the occurrence of late-stage disease/mortality are taken into account (Weiss, 1994). Factors can be related to the occurrence of late-stage disease by virtue of their relationship to disease incidence per se or to the likelihood of disease progression or spread. Thus, in a study of BSE and late-stage breast cancer, it would be necessary to evaluate (and possibly adjust for) characteristics that are associated with breast cancer incidence (e.g., race and educational level) and that differ between cases and controls. Similarly, adjustment would have to be made if women who regularly performed BSE also more commonly received the benefit of other detection methods for breast cancer (e.g., mammography and clinical examination) if the analysis found these other methods to have been efficacious (Weiss et al., 2004).

Questions

3.1. Pregnant women infected with *Trichomonas vaginalis* are at increased risk of premature delivery. A study of the efficacy of antibiotic treatment for this condition (Klebanoff et al., 2001) screened 31,157 asymptomatic women in the second trimester of pregnancy and, of the 2,377 found to be infected with *T. vaginalis*, randomly assigned 617 to receive two 2-gram doses of metronidazole or a placebo. Resolution of the infection was more common in the treatment group than in women who received a placebo (92.6% vs. 35.4%). However, if anything, preterm delivery occurred relatively more commonly in women assigned to take metronidazole (19.0% vs. 10.7%).

You have a patient in her 15th week of pregnancy who has no vaginal symptoms. What implications do the results of the study by Klebanoff et al. have on your decision to screen her for *T. vaginalis* infection?

3.2. The 5-year survival of men with localized cancer of the prostate gland is about 60%, whereas the 5-year survival of men with regional involvement from this disease is about 50%. A new test has been developed that, if applied in asymptomatic men, will enable all cases to be diagnosed at the localized stage. The test is inexpensive and innocuous. The developers of the test claim that if the test is used in asymptomatic men, mortality rates from prostate cancer will decrease. What reservations do you have regarding this claim?

3.3. A randomized trial has been conducted of the ability of electronic home monitoring of uterine contractions to reduce the risk of prematurity. Pregnant women at high risk of delivering prematurely (based on a history of a prior premature birth or on the presence of twins in the current pregnancy) were assigned at random to be monitored or not to be monitored, all other obstetric care being the same in the two groups. The women were followed for the development of preterm labor, defined as the presence of ≥ 4 contractions per hour plus a change in the cervix from a previous examination.

Among those with preterm labor, the mean time to delivery was 3.7 weeks in the monitored group and 2.0 weeks in the unmonitored group. This observed difference was unlikely to be due to chance in the absence of a true difference associated with monitoring.

Do these results necessarily indicate that electronic home uterine monitoring of high-risk pregnant women leads to a reduced incidence of prematurity?

Answers

3.1. If there is no benefit to be gained from recognizing the presence of *T. vaginalis* infection in an asymptomatic, pregnant woman, there is no purpose in making an effort to recognize it. The results of Klebanoff et al. argue that treating such infections with metronidazole will not reduce the incidence of premature delivery and, indeed, may increase that incidence. Only if an alternative therapy that actually is efficacious becomes available, or if there is some other benefit to be gained from knowledge of a *T. vaginalis* infection, could screening for this organism during pregnancy be recommended.

3.2. It is not necessarily true that mortality rates from carcinoma of the prostate will diminish following implementation of the new test. From the data presented, we do not even know whether it is more advantageous to diagnose a case of prostate cancer at the localized stage than at the regional stage. The difference in 5-year survival between the two groups, 60% versus 50%, could conceivably be due to lead-time bias. Second, we are unable to tell from these data whether the cases previously diagnosed at the regional stage would have had a better prognosis if they had been diagnosed at the localized stage. It may be that these are men with inherently more aggressive tumors that, irrespective of stage at diagnosis, would produce high mortality. The evaluation of the efficacy of the new test in reducing mortality rates from prostate cancer requires one of the following two approaches: (a) a one-step study in which groups of men who do and do not receive the test are monitored for their mortality rate from prostate cancer from the time of testing or (b) a comparison of the survival of treated and untreated men found to have localized cancer as a result of the test.

3.3. It is necessary to ask, Could the observed results—a 1.7-week difference in time to delivery favoring the monitored group—have occurred if no effective treatment had been available for the early preterm labor that monitoring would identify? Because of the possibility of lead-time bias, the answer is yes—among women who develop preterm labor, those in the monitored group will be identified earlier during the course of labor (to the extent that this test does achieve early detection), and so the interval from the *measured* onset of labor until delivery will be longer in them.

The appropriate analysis of the efficacy of a randomized trial of electronic home uterine monitoring would not be restricted to the women with premature labor. Rather, that analysis would compare the proportion of all women in each of the two groups (monitored, unmonitored) who develop an adverse outcome (e.g., premature delivery).

References

Bucher HC, Schmidt J. Does routine ultrasound scanning improve outcome in pregnancy? Meta-analysis of various outcome measures. *Br Med J* 1993;307:13–16.

Buekens P, Alexander S, Boutsen M, et al. European Community Collaborative Study Group on Prenatal Screening: Randomized controlled trial of routine cervical examinations in pregnancy. *Lancet* 1994;344:841–844.

Cornfield J. A method of estimating comparative rates from clinical data: Applications to cancer of the lung, breast, and cervix. *J Natl Cancer Inst* 1951;11:1269–1275.

Dronfield MW, McIllmurray MB, Ferguson R, et al. A prospective, randomized study of endoscopy and radiology in acute upper-gastrointestinal-tract bleeding. *Lancet* 1977;1:1167–1169.

Early Treatment Diabetic Retinopathy Study Research Group. Treatment techniques and clinical guidelines for photocoagulation of diabetic macular edema. *Ophthalmology* 1987; 94:761–774.

Ewigman BG, Crane JP, Frigoletto FD, et al. Effect of prenatal ultrasound screening on perinatal outcome. RADIUS Study Group. *N Engl J Med* 1993;329:821–827.

Gibson NA, Hollman AS, Paton JY. Value of radiological follow up of child-hood pneumonia. *Br Med J* 1993;307:1117.

Hanley JA, Lippman-Hand A. If nothing goes wrong, is everything all right? Interpreting zero numerators. *JAMA* 1983;249:1743–1745.

Johannesson G, Geirsson G, Day N. The effect of mass screening in Iceland, 1965–74 on the incidence and mortality of cervical carcinoma. *Int J Cancer* 1978;21:418–425.

Klebanoff MA, Carey JC, Hauth JC, et al. Failure of metronidazole to pre-vent preterm delivery among pregnant women with asymptomatic *Trichomonas vaginalis* infection. *N Engl J Med* 2001;345:487–493.

Kramer MS, Mills EL, MacLellan AM, et al. Effects of obtaining a blood cul-ture on subsequent management of young febrile children without an ev-ident focus of infection. *Can Med Assoc J* 1986;135:1125–1129.

Mahomed K, Nyoni R, Mulambo T, et al. Randomised controlled trial of in-trapartum fetal heart rate monitoring. *Br Med J* 1994;308:497–500.

Mandel JS, Bond JH, Church TR, et al. Reducing mortality from colorectal cancer by screening for fecal occult blood. *N Engl J Med* 1993;328:1365–1371.

Morrison AS. Case definition in case-control studies of the efficacy of screen-ing. *Am J Epidemiol* 1982;115:6–8.

Moss SE, Klein R, Kessler SD, et al. Comparison between ophthalmoscopy and fundus photography in determining severity of diabetic retinopathy. *Ophthalmology* 1985;92:62–67.

Multicentre Aneurysm Screening Study Group. The Multicentre Aneurysm Screening Study (MASS) into the effect of abdominal aortic aneurysm screening on mortality in men: A randomised controlled trial. *Lancet* 2002;360:1531–1539.

Neutra RR, Fienberg SE, Greenland S, et al. Effect of fetal monitoring on neonatal death rates. *N Engl J Med* 1978;299:324–326.

Schwartz RH, Wientzen RL. Occult bacteremia in toxic-appearing, febrile infants. *Clin Pediatr* 1982;21:659–663.

Shapiro S, Venet W, Strax P, et al. Ten- to fourteen-year effect of screening on breast cancer mortality. *J Natl Cancer Inst* 1982;69:349–355.

Teele DW, Pelton SI, Grant MJ, et al. Bacteremia in febrile children under 2 years of age: Results in cultures of blood of 600 consecutive febrile chil-dren seen in a "walk-in" clinic. *Pediatrics* 1975;87:227–230.

Thomas DB, Gao DL, Ray RM, et al. Randomized trial of breast self-examination in Shanghai: Final results. *J Natl Cancer Inst* 2002;94:1445–1457.

US Preventive Services Task Force. Home uterine activity monitoring for preterm labor. *JAMA* 1993;270:371–376.

Weiss NS. Control definition in case-control studies of the efficacy of screen-ing and diagnostic testing. *Am J Epidemiol* 1983;118:457–460.

Weiss NS. Application of the case-control method in the evaluation of screen-ing. *Epidemiol Rev* 1994;16:102–108.

Weiss NS, McKnight B, Stevens NG. Approaches to the analysis of case-control studies of the efficacy of screening for cancer. *Am J Epidemiol* 1992;135:817–823.

Weiss NS, Dhillon PK, Etzioni R. Case-control studies of the efficacy of cancer screening: Overcoming bias from non-random patterns of screening. *Epidemiology* 2004;15:409–413.

Zelen M. Theory of early detection of breast cancer in the general population, in Heusen JC, Mattheim WH, Rozencweig M, eds. *Breast Cancer: Trends in Research and Treatment.* New York: Raven Press; 1976.

4

Therapeutic Efficacy

Randomized Controlled Trials

A randomized controlled trial of therapeutic efficacy is one in which (a) patients are assigned to one of two or more groups to be offered different therapeutic measures, (b) chance alone dictates whether a particular patient will be assigned to a particular group, and (c) patients in each group are monitored for the abatement of their illness or for the occurrence of the event(s) that the therapy seeks to prevent. Most randomized controlled trials provide results that can be interpreted relatively easily, for the common concern in nonrandomized studies—that the various treatment groups had inherently unequal probabilities of doing well—is much less pressing when it is only chance that determines the membership of the groups. The popularity of randomized trials has increased during the past several decades. The approach has been applied to virtually every class of therapy, from pharmaceutical agents to surgical techniques to dietary and other "lifestyle" interventions.

The concept of a randomized controlled trial is straightforward. However, a number of issues that are not so straightforward have to be considered when planning the design and analysis of a particular study. The ways in which these issues are dealt with often have a substantial bearing on the validity and interpretation of the results.

Choosing the Subjects for Study

Generalizing beyond the Study Population

The rationale for research in clinical epidemiology is that by observing the illness experience of some persons we may come away with lessons that can be applied more broadly. So, by determining that persons randomly assigned to receive drug A fare better than those assigned to receive drug B, we can conclude that persons similar to those in the study will do better on the average by taking drug A rather than drug B.

To what extent must these two groups—study subjects and persons to whom we would like to refer the findings (reference population)—be "similar" so that valid generalizations can be made from one to the other? To answer this question, it is necessary to take into account the answers to two other questions: (a) Do both the study and reference populations suffer untoward consequences from the condition for which the therapy is being given? (b) If the therapy is effective in the study population, would the means by which it is believed to act (i.e., its biological effect) be present in members of the reference population as well?

To illustrate how the issue of generalizing is approached in practice, let's place ourselves back in the late 1960s, immediately following the publication of the results of the first large randomized controlled trial of antihypertensive therapy for the reduction of mortality from cardiovascular disease (Veterans Administration Cooperative Study Group on Antihypertensive Agents, 1967). The study documented a substantial mortality reduction in actively treated versus placebo-treated male veterans with a diastolic blood pressure of 115 to 129 mm Hg who were free of clinical cardiac or cerebrovascular disease and in whom there was no advanced retinal or renal pathology. Now let's say we had a patient with that level of blood pressure who was neither a veteran nor male. Should we presume that the findings apply to her? Is a randomized trial of the efficacy of antihypertensive drugs needed in nonveteran women? We would address the issue by considering, first, whether high blood pressure in nonveterans and women predisposes them to an increased risk of mortality from cardiovascular diseases. In 1967, data were available indicating that such persons indeed were at increased risk. (Of course, there are other situations in which the available data suggest no parallel relationship. For example, in middle-aged persons mortality from cardiovascular disease is positively associated with levels of serum cholesterol, but this is not so among the elderly [Kronmal et al., 1993]. Also, it may be that data that link the condition with the outcome just are not available for the population or disease subgroup to which a patient belongs.)

Second, we would ask whether the postulated mechanism through which antihypertensive therapy exerted its beneficial effect on mortality in male veterans is present in nonveteran women. Unfortunately, it is rarely possible to arrive at an unequivocal answer to a question of this sort, for our knowledge of the means by which the therapy works is rarely definitive. Although there would be no basis for believing that nonveterans differ from veterans in this respect, it is not out of the question that hormonal and other differences between the sexes could make the extrapolation from men to women inexact. The uncertainty would likely be greater still when trying to extrapolate the study results to persons with diastolic blood pressure levels below 115 mm Hg. The benefit of antihypertensive therapy would be expected to be smaller in these persons (for their excess risk is smaller), but by how much? This is no minor matter, as there are more people with modest elevations of blood pressure than there are with large elevations, and a blood pressure threshold must be set below which therapy will not be instituted.[1]

In general, unless we can identify a characteristic of a patient (e.g., age, gender, nationality) that we have good reason to believe would influence the efficacy of a therapy, we ought to be willing to apply lessons learned from randomized trials conducted in patients without that characteristic. Of course, what is a "good reason" to some will not be to others, and disagreements in this area can be expected to arise. Perhaps a relatively greater degree of caution should be used when seeking to generalize the results of one or more randomized trials of a therapy for a given severity or manifestation of an illness to patients with a different severity or manifestation. The reduced mortality from cardiovascular disease that has been demonstrated in randomized trials of pharmacologic treatment of diastolic blood pressures of 100 mm Hg or more does not mean there will necessarily be any benefit if the same treatment is given to persons whose diastolic pressure is 85 mm Hg (Siscovick et al., 1996). The administration of a monoclonal antibody against a surface glycoprotein of epithelial cells appears to improve survival of patients with colorectal cancer and lymph node spread who have undergone successful surgical resection of all visible tumor (Riethmuller et al., 1994). However, these results may not be applicable to other patients with metastatic colorectal tumors, given the more substantial barriers to the delivery of monoclonal antibodies in patients with a relatively larger tumor burden (Jain, 1990).

Maximizing the Study's Ability to Identify Therapeutic Efficacy

Some leap of faith is going to have to be made in applying the results obtained in the study subjects to the reference population. Therefore, the choice of the particular group of subjects for study often depends less on the degree

---

[1] By the end of the 1970s, randomized trials had demonstrated the efficacy of antihypertensive therapy in nonveterans, women, and persons with less extreme blood pressure elevation (Hypertension Detection and Follow-Up Program Cooperative Group, 1979a,b).

to which the group represents the reference population than on the group's having characteristics that will produce a study that will successfully identify a difference between treatments if one is truly present. There are 2 such important characteristics.

Low Cost of Enrolling and Monitoring Members of the Group

The lower the cost per subject, the larger will be the number of subjects available at a given budget level (it is necessary to get these studies funded!), and the more statistically powerful will be the study. An early investigation of the effect of a low-cholesterol, low-saturated-fat diet on the incidence of cardiovascular disease was conducted in a Veterans Administration psychiatric hospital (Dayton et al., 1969). Patients receiving meals from one kitchen had a modified diet, whereas the diet of other patients remained as before. The cost of performing this intervention at an institution clearly was less than that of trying to modify dietary cholesterol and saturated fat on an individual basis in individual kitchens.

Once a group of investigators has been established to conduct a randomized controlled trial, there is an economy in having these same investigators conduct additional studies. The initial administrative costs (and possibly also the costs that can be associated with the group's early inexperience) can be avoided when another therapy for the disease is to be evaluated or when the investigators evaluate a therapy for another disease that they encounter. In some instances, the same patients enrolled and participating in the first study can be enrolled in the second study. For example, to determine whether aspirin use could prevent myocardial infarction, participants in some treatment groups of the Coronary Drug Project that had been disbanded (e.g., those assigned to receive estrogen or thyroid hormones) but who were still under surveillance were randomly assigned to receive aspirin or placebo (Coronary Drug Project Research Group, 1976).

High Expected Compliance with the Therapeutic Regimens

Many randomized trials begin with a "run-in" phase in which all potential subjects are given a placebo or a "control" therapy. Their compliance with the regimen is assessed, and only those in whom compliance is good are entered into the randomized portion of the study (also see p. 56). This is yet another assault on the "representativeness" of the study subjects vis-à-vis other populations, for the latter invariably would include volunteers and nonvolunteers, compliers and noncompliers, to whom one would like to extrapolate the results. Yet the resulting study population offers a "clean" separation of subjects exposed to the various treatments and thus enhances the ability to find any true between-treatment difference that might exist.

Nonetheless, there is the occasional study that has as its goal the measurement of the impact of an intervention in a population to whom the intervention is offered, that is, the efficacy in those who receive it *combined with* the dilution that results from whatever noncompliance exists in that population. For example, the study of mammography and clinical breast examination conducted within the Health Insurance Plan of New York randomly assigned some of the female members to the intervention group and only then notified them of the study (Shapiro et al., 1971). A sizable fraction of these women, 35%, failed to attend even a single screening examination. Nonetheless, the aim of the study was to determine whether screening of this type would reduce mortality from breast cancer in a population to whom it was offered—not the efficacy of screening, narrowly defined, but its real-world "effectiveness" (Last, 1995). This aim was served fully by comparing mortality in the study group, at whatever level of compliance, with that of other women in the Plan.

Nature of the Intervention

Generalizing beyond the Therapeutic Measure under Study

Often a number of interventions can accomplish the same biochemical or physiologic change. Arterial blood pressure, for example, can be reduced in a variety of ways. If only one of the therapies has been evaluated (say, against a placebo) and a beneficial effect has been found in preventing or controlling a clinical manifestation that results from the original biochemical/physiological derangement, what can be said of the benefits expected from the use of another therapy that is believed to rectify the derangement through another means?

Here, just as with the question of generalizing from the study to the reference population, it is not possible to provide a definitive answer that covers all situations. To the extent that the means by which the evaluated therapy exerted its beneficial effect is (a) known and (b) shared by the not-yet-evaluated therapy, there will be confidence that the latter is also effective. However, because this is a subjective assessment, not all who review the evidence will arrive at the same conclusion.

> *Example:* A decline in mortality from coronary disease was noted in persons assigned at random to take cholestyramine, an agent that alters the concentration of certain serum lipids (Lipid Research Clinics Program, 1983). Would it be reasonable to assume that a diet that can accomplish similar changes in lipid levels will accomplish a similar reduction in mortality? Initially, it might have been reasonable to be cautious in trying to answer this question, as one could speculate that the metabolic effect of cholestyramine that is relevant to coronary disease is not shared by a low-saturated-fat, low-cholesterol diet. Nonethe-

less, the subsequent documentation of the beneficial effect on coronary disease progression of partial ileal bypass surgery (Buchwald et al., 1990), yet another method of producing the same types of serum lipid alterations, argued that such a diet would be effective, as well. By the same reasoning, at the time of the introduction of statins into practice, there was a basis for believing that use of these drugs should lower the incidence of and mortality from coronary heart disease, given that their favorable influence on levels of serum lipids had been documented to be quite strong. However, statins can have multiple biologic effects, and it was important that randomized trials of statins be conducted to determine the net effect (across all mechanisms) of their use on coronary disease. The results of these studies suggest a favorable impact of statins that begins relatively soon after treatment has begun (Stenestrand et al., 2001; Shepherd et al., 2002) and that is not restricted to persons with serum lipid abnormalities (Long-Term Intervention with Pravastatin in Ischaemic Disease Study Group, 1998). This pattern of results argues that lipid lowering may not be the only means by which statin use produces its clinical benefits.

Maximizing the Study's Ability to Identify Therapeutic Efficacy

Suppose you are evaluating the effect of dietary modification on disease, say a diet low in saturated fat in relation to the occurrence of myocardial infarction. It would be important to make the modified diet as different as possible from that of persons in the control arm of the study, within the range of what is ethical to recommend and what you believe will be acceptable to patients. If it is only below a certain threshold of saturated fat intake that an impact on myocardial infarction is evident, you would like the intake of participants in the intervention arm of your study to be below that threshold. Alternatively, the relation of saturated fat intake to the incidence of myocardial infarction could be a graded one. If so, the greater the disparity of saturated fat intake between participants in the intervention and control arms of the study, the greater will be the size of the association (on average), and therefore the greater the ability of the study to observe an impact on the risk of myocardial infarction.

Occasionally, investigators substitute an artificial intervention to maximize the difference in exposure status between treatment and control groups. For example, in an attempt to measure the role of sodium intake on blood pressure in persons with mild hypertension (Australian National Health and Medical Research Council Dietary Salt Study Management Committee, 1989), patients instructed to adopt a diet containing less than 80 mmol sodium per day were randomized to receive: (a) 80 mmol sodium chloride per day, in the form of 8 slow-release tablets; or (b) 8 placebo tablets daily. It is likely that the substantial between-group difference in sodium ingestion produced by this design contributed to the clear differences in blood pressure seen during the 8-week follow-up period.

Should More Than One Intervention Be Included in the Same Randomized Trial?

Because of the limited statistical power of many trials to document clinically important differences between two therapeutic regimens, the decision to add an evaluation of one or more other therapies must not be made lightly. There can be strong temptations to form additional treatment groups. There may be several promising therapies, or there may be some uncertainty as to the proper dose/duration of a single therapy, and it might seem advantageous to try several. For example, after a randomized trial in which aspirin was found not to lower the risk of recurrence in persons with a previous myocardial infarction (Aspirin Myocardial Infarction Study Research Group, 1980), it was suggested that a beneficial effect might have been present had only a different dose of aspirin been used (Lorenz et al., 1984). Nonetheless, obtaining an adequate number of subjects assigned to receive a particular treatment regimen so that there can be a valid test of at least one hypothesis should remain the first priority.

If two (or more) therapies are believed to influence the consequences or progression of a disease but not to do so jointly through a single biological mechanism, it is reasonable to include each one in a single randomized trial that uses a *factorial* design. If there were 2 therapies, A and B, such a design would involve the formation of 4 treatment groups based on the receipt of A alone, B alone, A + B, or neither treatment. The assessment of the effect of treatment A would involve 2 comparisons: A alone versus no treatment and A+B versus B alone. If the 2 comparisons provided the same result, they could be aggregated to give an overall indication of A's effect.

Factorial designs have the potential to answer questions regarding the efficacy of several possible treatments in a relatively efficient way (Byar et al., 1993). However, because of the possibility that the impact of therapy A differs depending on whether therapy B is also given, and vice versa, presentation of the experience of each of the separate treatment groups in the trial is necessary in order for the results to be correctly interpreted (Lubsen and Pocock, 1994).

Nature of the Therapy to Be Administered to the Comparison Group

Typically, the comparison group is prescribed "conventional" therapy, which may range from no therapy at all to a complex array of interventions that is believed, at the time the trial is being planned, to be the best that can be offered. To justify the conduct of the study, of course, equipoise must be present, that is, a state of uncertainty as to which among the alternative treatment options being considered for inclusion in the potential trial is superior. Thus there should be a nearly identical probability that the comparison therapy, even if it is no therapy, will prove to be as good as or superior to the therapy under study (Freedman, 1987). A judgment as to what is "nearly identical" will be based on existing data, usually from nonrandomized studies. Because a judgment is involved, there often will be disagreement among investigators as to the adequacy of these data in determining the efficacy of the therapy being considered for study, and thus there often will be disagreement as to whether it is ethical to subject some patients to the conventional (or to the new) therapy (Stein and Pincus, 1999; Ellenberg and Temple, 2000); Emanuel and Miller, 2001).

If some form of placebo is to be used, it should be, if possible, totally innocuous. However, in some situations the manipulation necessary to administer the therapy is such that, in the absence of a similar manipulation in the comparison group, the internal validity of the study could be undermined due to a placebo effect. Thus, in a study of the efficacy of auricular acupuncture in the treatment of cocaine addiction (Margolin et al., 2002), patients were randomly assigned to have 4 needles inserted: (a) in or near the concha (the treatment hypothesized to be of benefit); or (b) in the helis of the auricle (the "control" arm of the trial). However, as the nature of the control intervention becomes increasingly invasive, ethical issues loom increasingly large. For example, consider the randomized trial by Carette et al. (1997) to evaluate the effect of an epidural injection of methylprednisolone acetate to relieve sciatica due to a herniated lumbar disc. A needle was placed into the epidural space of each study subject, who was then given either the steroid or sterile saline on a random basis. The administration of an epidural injection of an inert substance could never be considered a legitimate therapeutic alternative—it poses at least some risk and discomfort to the patient with little or no possibility of benefit—so how can it be justified ethically? The only way is to inform the prospective subjects as to the nature of the study and of the rationale for the use of a placebo that is not free of risk and/or discomfort. They can then decide whether they are willing to subject themselves to the risks so that others may benefit from the higher quality of information the trial can thereby provide.

Randomized controlled trials of coronary artery bypass surgery have eschewed the use of blinding by means of a "sham" surgical procedure and have instead assigned comparison patients to "medical" therapy (Principal Investigators of CASS and Associates, 1981). The choice of comparison patients in whom no surgery was performed meant that study participants and their caregivers were not blinded to allocation status and thus that certain important research questions could not be unambiguously addressed. Specifically, it would be impossible to determine whether any reduced level of pain in the patients undergoing bypass surgery, relative to that in the medical therapy group, was a result of the bypass per se or simply of the more general effect of a surgical procedure performed within the chest (Cobb et al., 1959). Nonetheless, it would have been inappropriate to do anything other than place the patients' welfare first, even though that forced some of the goals of the studies to be compromised.

Clearly, this lack of blinding of subjects and investigators will prove more important in the interpretation of some outcomes (e.g., chest pain) than of others (e.g., mortality). If possible, of course, it is better to keep both subjects and investigators ignorant of the treatment status, as this will minimize the possibility of actions on the part of either group that could bias the results. When complications of disease or therapy arise that necessitate knowledge of the specific therapy to which the patient has been assigned, this information usually can be given to one or more physicians external to the study who can decide on the proper course of action. If the therapy under study is a drug, the blinding is generally done by preparing a placebo identical in appearance to the active agent. However, one study in which the identical appearance of drug and placebo was achieved but blinding was not is instructive to review here:

> *Example:* In the early 1970s, healthy adults were enrolled in a randomized controlled trial in which they were asked to take vitamin C (3 g/day) or a lactose placebo for 9 months, during which time the incidence of colds was monitored (Karlowski et al., 1975). Because some subjects indicated that they had bitten into and tasted the preparation that they had been given, the investigators asked all subjects at the conclusion of the study to guess the group to which they had been assigned. Of the 102 who attempted a guess, 79 were correct (77%). Eleven percent more of the subjects given a placebo had 2 or more colds during the follow-up period than did those given vitamin C. However, an even larger difference was associated with a subject's believing he or she was assigned to a particular group: 36% of subjects assigned to receive vitamin C had 2 or more colds, twice the incidence in persons who, though they actually were taking placebo, thought they were taking vitamin C. A similar difference was found for persons who received the vitamin but believed it was a placebo—the proportion of this group with 2 or more colds was higher than that among persons receiving placebo (67% vs. 47%). Because a subject's suspicion of the group to which he or she had been assigned so strongly influenced the results, and because a subject's suspicion was much more often right than wrong, the validity of the vitamin C-placebo comparison was seriously compromised.

Among those 2-arm randomized trials in which no untreated or placebo group is included, there are some in which the goal is to determine whether the treatments being compared are equally effective. This goal may be sought once one of the treatments has been shown to be effective and when a second treatment—not yet similarly evaluated—has potential advantages in terms of ease of administration, cost, or the incidence of adverse effects. In such "equivalence" studies, a conclusion that the 2 treatments work to the same degree can be made if the confidence interval surrounding the difference in the observed efficacy entirely lies within some prespecified range that corresponds to there being no material clinical difference. So suppose, for example, that treatment A were associated with "improvement" in 69% of patients and treatment B in 67% and that the 95% confidence interval around the difference of 2% were −3 to +7 percent. If it were felt that equivalence corresponded to a true difference of <10% between the treatments, then the results of the trial would be deemed to be compatible with equivalence.

"Equivalence" studies generally need to enroll a large number of patients. Without a large number, the confidence interval surrounding even an observed absence of difference will be too wide to exclude a true between-treatment difference in efficacy of an important size. These studies also need to achieve a high level of compliance; without this, an observation of similar results between patients assigned to each of the 2 treatments will have little credibility, as the impact of noncompliance is almost always to produce a spuriously low estimate of any true differences in efficacy (see p. 67). Further details of the design, analysis, and potential limitations of "equivalence" studies can be found in Jones et al. (1996) and Temple and Ellenberg (2000).

Assignment of Subjects to Treatment Groups

How Should the Assignment Be Made?

The method of patient assignment should guarantee that chance alone dictates the allocation of a particular patient to a particular treatment group. The available means of accomplishing this are described elsewhere (Rosenberger and Lachin, 2002, pp. 155–161). The health professional involved in the patient's care, having made the decision to ask him or her to participate in the study, should have no role in the assignment process. It is necessary to safeguard against letting the provider's judgment concerning which patient needs or does not need the therapy under study influence the treatment assignment.

When Should the Random Assignment Take Place?

In most randomized controlled trials, subjects are assigned to the treatment groups only after they have been informed of the nature of the study and of the therapies they may be offered. For example, in the trial designed to evaluate the efficacy of coronary artery bypass surgery (Principal Investigators of CASS and Associates, 1981), patients who were deemed eligible for surgery—but not those in whom surgery was deemed essential—were asked to allow themselves to be assigned at random to receive either the surgery or the medical therapy. The study included only those patients who agreed to submit to the luck of the draw. See Figure 4.1 for a schematic representation of this approach.

There are some circumstances, however, in which it might be advisable to make the random assignment prior to requesting participation:

1. The investigator and/or clinical collaborators may be uncomfortable with the idea of presenting the possibility of a choice of therapy to a patient. In the case of a life-threatening illness (e.g., cancer), perhaps the investigator is concerned that patients not assigned to the newest, most radical measures may withdraw from the trial, even after consent has been given, in order to actively seek these treatments. In such a circumstance, the investigator can randomly assign patients to alternative therapies and either (a) seek consent to participate in the study from all patients, whether they have been assigned the standard or the new therapy (Ellenberg, 1984), or (b) seek consent only from patients assigned the new therapy (Zelen, 1979). Zelen (1990) has discussed the ethical and practical issues that can arise in studies of this type.
2. Sometimes the efficacy of an intervention is to be studied within a large, defined group of individuals (e.g., members of a prepaid health care plan) who have not actively sought care from the investigative team. This situation might arise in an evaluation of vaccine efficacy in healthy individuals or of a screening technique for cancer. In such situations, it could prove logistically difficult and unnecessarily costly to contact and explain the study to all persons rather than to just the fraction to whom the intervention measure will be offered.

A trial that randomizes participants prior to seeking consent will be limited in its attempt to assess treatment efficacy if a high proportion of subjects to whom the treatment is offered choose not to accept it. The reason is that patients who refuse the treatment will, in the primary analysis of data gathered in the trial, be retained in the same group as those who comply. Therefore, a low level of compliance will obscure any true treatment-related benefit.

In the "conventional" type of randomized trial (i.e., agreement to participate prior to randomization), it may be desirable to postpone randomization of a patient until his or her compliance can be evaluated (assuming noncompliance is a possibility, e.g., in a drug or lifestyle intervention study). The measurement of compliance can take many forms (pill counts, biochemical tests, etc.), but the goal is the same: to eliminate before the start of the study patients who have a high likelihood of not adhering to the regimen offered and who are therefore likely to be a source of misclassification within the study. With this issue in mind, the study of the value of lowering blood pressure conducted within the Veterans Administration (Veterans Administration Cooperative Study Group on Antihypertensive Agents, 1967) administered to all eligible hypertensive subjects a placebo tablet that contained 5 mg of riboflavin for 2 to 4 months. Because the urine of persons who take

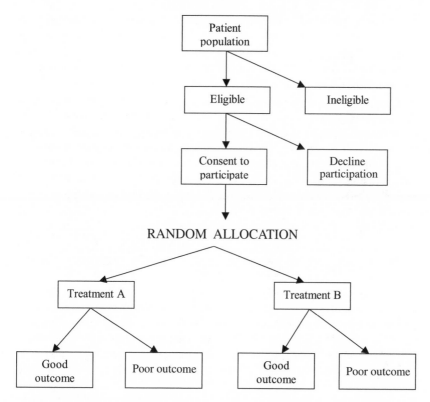

Figure 4.1 Schematic representation of a trial using random allocation of patients to treatment groups.

riboflavin is fluorescent yellow under ultraviolet light, the investigators had an objective measure of compliance available only to them. Only those subjects whose compliance achieved a designated level—a bare majority of the potential subjects—were enrolled in that randomized trial of antihypertensive agents.

Under What Circumstances Can a Subject Serve as His or Her Own Control?

There are many conditions that affect more than one part of the body, and for some of these conditions it is possible to administer therapy locally that has no effect on untreated lesions elsewhere. In such a situation, it is appropriate to design a study so that one or more lesions are randomly selected for treatment, with others serving as control sites. Such a design has been used to evaluate measures intended to control diabetic retinopathy (Diabetic Retinopathy Study Research Group, 1981) and some dermatologic conditions (Gilchrest et al., 1979).

Studies of the efficacy of therapies intended to reduce the frequency or severity of chronic, recurrent problems, such as seizures, arthritic pain, or menopausal hot flashes, can be more precise in a statistical sense if the subject can serve as his or her own control. By evaluating the same subject at different times, in the presence and the absence of the therapy under study, the variability among subjects in the frequency or severity of the problem will not blur true differences in efficacy. This can be achieved experimentally in a "crossover" design, in which the study subjects are divided into 2 groups and dealt with as shown in Figure 4.2. For each of some number of subjects, the primary comparison is between the frequency and/or severity of the condition during (or at the end of) the time intervals 0–1 and 2–3 (Hills and Armitage, 1979). Events occurring during the period between time points 1 and 2, the length of which is determined largely by the amount of time needed for the effects of the measures initially administered to dissipate, are not included in the analysis. (Crossover studies are not appropriate for evaluating the efficacy of therapeutic measures whose effects following discontinuation do not dissipate relatively quickly, i.e., within several days.)

In crossover studies it is important to include both sequences, therapy-control and control-therapy, for the effect of the therapy can be confounded by the sequence in which it is given (Louis et al., 1984). An example of what could happen if only 1 sequence were used can be seen in a crossover study of estrogen versus placebo for the relief of symptoms associated with menopause (Coope et al., 1975). Women entering the study averaged 50 to 60 episodes of hot flashes per week. In the group assigned to receive placebo first, the rate fell to 20 per week after 3 months and fell further, to less than 5 per week, at the end of a subsequent 3-month period on estrogen therapy. So, in women who started with placebo and crossed over to estrogens, there was evidence of efficacy of estrogen use, although not of an overly great magnitude relative to the "efficacy" of a placebo. It was in the group of women assigned to the other sequence—estrogen first, placebo second—that a large difference occurred. After 3 months on estrogens the frequency of hot flashes fell to less than 5 per week, but the switch to placebo resulted in a return to the original 50 to 60 per week. Although the reasons for the difference in measured efficacy between the 2 sequences are not well understood, the fact that such a difference can occur reinforces the idea that both possible sequences in a crossover study must be examined.

Although most crossover studies employ 1 treatment and 1 control period in each of a group of patients, it is also possible to do studies of single patients in which there are multiple periods, randomly chosen, of a treatment and a control intervention (Guyatt et al., 1986; McLeod et al., 1986). The analysis of such an "N of 1" study would compare the overall experience of the patient, commonly the presence or degree of symptoms the therapy is intended to prevent or ameliorate, during (or at the conclusion of) the treatment and control intervals. Studies of this sort can be particularly useful in drawing inferences regarding the efficacy of therapy in the individual patient(s) studied, though

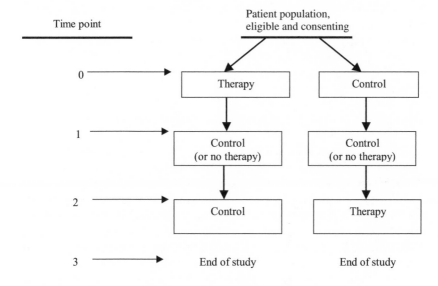

Figure 4.2 Schematic representation of trial using a crossover design.

relatively less so in judging how much, if any, benefit other patients would receive from that same therapy.

Assessment of Endpoints in Study Subjects

There should be standard criteria by which study endpoints can be assessed, preferably stipulated at the start of the trial. And, if possible, the person (or persons) who applies the criteria to a particular study participant should be ignorant of the treatment group to which that participant has been assigned.

Incomplete follow-up of study participants for the development of outcome events is a threat to the validity of the results of a randomized trial. This is a particular concern for trials in which the assessment of outcomes requires an examination or interview during the follow-up period. For example, in a randomized study of a pharmacologic intervention for depression, persons receiving the drug under investigation and those assigned to nonpharmacologic therapy might be compared (after a number of weeks) for the presence of suicidal ideation. If attrition from the study is appreciable and differs between persons with and without such ideation and also differs between persons assigned to drug and nondrug therapy, the efficacy of the drug will be inaccurately measured.

The specific means of enhancing completeness of follow-up will depend on the circumstances of the study setting and study population. However, the vigor with which members of the treatment groups are followed must be equivalent, so that the detection of any study endpoints that do occur is comparable among groups.

Comparison of the Treatment Groups for the Occurrence of Endpoints

Which Endpoints to Count

In planning most randomized controlled trials, the choice of endpoint is clear. A study of an analgesic would measure the patient's perception of pain; a study of an antibiotic would measure the disappearance of infection and its clinical manifestations. However, some therapies have such a high potential for serious adverse effects that a broad range of endpoints must be considered. In a randomized trial of the efficacy of transplantation in prolonging life, it would not make sense to look at mortality rates in transplanted and nontransplanted patients only for the cause of death at which the therapy was directed (e.g., renal failure, leukemia). Rather, it would be necessary to count causes of death that are related to rejection of the transplant as well. In practice, one probably would tabulate all causes of death combined.

In many studies, the primary outcome of interest is the occurrence of 2 or more events that are believed to be different manifestations of the same underlying disease process. For example, the central analysis of a randomized trial conducted among patients with acute ischemic heart disease might compare those in the treated and control arms for the occurrence of any of the following: death, myocardial infarction, or refractory ischemia. A trial conducted in patients with primary sclerosing cholangitis considered a composite outcome, the components of which were death, liver transplantation, or one of several indicators of deterioration of hepatic function (Lindor et al., 1997). If the occurrence of each of the components of one of these aggregate outcome definitions truly is influenced to the same degree by the intervention measure, then the study will benefit from having a greater level of statistical precision than a study focusing on the separate outcomes one at a time. However, if the impact of the intervention is not uniform on all components, the interpretation of the study results may not be straightforward (Freemantle et al., 2003).

In studies with mortality as an endpoint, a problem arises when the cause of death against which the therapy is directed does not constitute an overwhelming majority of the total deaths and yet no good information is available a priori as to which other causes might be affected. The problem exists because neither the rate of the specific cause of death nor the overall mortality rate is wholly satisfactory. A comparison based on all causes of death incorporates many extraneous endpoints, and so one runs the risk of diluting a true effect of the therapy and making it harder to identify (Church et al., 2002; Weiss and Koepsell, 2002). However, an analysis based on a single cause of death may provide only an incomplete picture of the therapy's effects. The interpretation of such a study may benefit from having both analyses done.

Example: A randomized controlled trial was conducted in which clofibrate or a placebo was given for an average of 5.3 years to hypercholesterolemic men in order to gauge the influence of clofibrate on the incidence and mortality of arteriosclerotic vascular disease (Committee of Principal Investigators, 1978). The rate of nonfatal myocardial infarction was decreased in the clofibrate-treated men, although the rate of fatal heart attack was similar in the 2 groups. However, other causes of death were more common in the treated group, particularly deaths from digestive diseases and cancer, so that the overall mortality in the clofibrate and placebo groups, respectively, was 2.2 and 1.7 per 1,000 per year. Had attention been restricted to the endpoint of myocardial infarction, important information about the effects of clofibrate would have been missed.

Some conditions that one is attempting to treat or prevent from occurring have measurable antecedents. For example, following treatment for cancer, a death from that cancer is usually preceded by tumor recurrence or metastasis. Death from suicide is often preceded by the presence of suicidal ideation. Because one of the factors limiting the power of a randomized trial is the number of endpoints, and because these antecedent conditions often occur more commonly than do the endpoints themselves, the monitoring and analysis of these antecedents ("surrogates") should increase the statistical power per subject enrolled.

As an investigator, you would be pleased to accept this increase in power as long as the analysis of the occurrence of such an antecedent condition provides, qualitatively, the same "answer" as would a study of a larger number of subjects in which the endpoint itself was measured. You will get the same answer to the extent that the occurrence of the antecedent condition is highly predictive of the endpoint:

Example: Following a myocardial infarction, many patients develop ventricular premature depolarizations (VPDs). Two drugs, encainide and flecainide, were developed that could offer at least partial protection against VPDs. To determine whether the use of these drugs could reduce mortality from cardiac arrhythmia, Echt et al. (1991) conducted a randomized controlled trial. Patients with >6 VPDs per hour after a recent myocardial infarction were treated for an average of 15 days with encainide or flecainide. Those who achieved >80% suppression of VPDs (some 75% of patients) were assigned either to continue one of the two drugs used or to receive a placebo. Among the 755 patients who received active treatment, 63 deaths occurred during the follow-up period, of which 43 were due to cardiac arrhythmia. The rate of each of these outcomes was about 2.5 times *higher* than that in the placebo groups. These unfortunate results, apart from arguing strongly against the continued use of encainide or flecainide in this clinical setting, tell us that suppression of VPDs is an inadequate measure of a drug's efficacy in preventing life-threatening arrhythmias.

Example: In order to access the efficacy of etidronate, an agent that reduces bone resorption by inhibiting osteoclastic activity, several studies (Storm et al., 1990; Watts et al., 1990; Adachi et al., 1997) randomly assigned postmenopausal osteoporotic women to receive the drug or a placebo for a 2- to 3-year period. In addition to monitoring bone density in the etidronate and control groups, the investigators also assessed the occurrence of vertebral fractures during the follow-up period. In all studies, the women who received etidronate had a greater bone density and a lower fracture rate than did women who received a placebo. Given the ability of another therapy for osteoporosis, fluoride, to improve bone density *without* lowering the rate of fracture (Riggs et al., 1990), the interpretation of the results of the etidronate studies is strengthened by the inclusion of fractures as an endpoint.

The following is another example of an intervention that was successful in modifying a suspected antecedent of an endpoint but that turned out to have no influence on the endpoint itself. It should serve to reinforce our caution in interpreting the results of randomized trials that measure a therapy's effect on an antecedent alone.

Example: To determine whether the incidence of hepatitis B infection could be reduced in persons undergoing long-term hemodialysis, a large, randomized controlled trial (*n* = 1,311) of hepatitis B vaccine was initiated (Stevens et al., 1984). Active production of antibody to hepatitis B surface antigen (anti-HBs) occurred in about 50% of the vaccinated group and in only 2% of those given a placebo. Nonetheless, during the 25-month follow-up period, the incidence of hepatitis B infection in the 2 groups was nearly identical. The authors concluded that "although anti-HBs is traditionally used as an index of immunity to [hepatitis B] infections, it may not be a crucial protective factor. . . . The vaccine we used may have failed to induce such protective responses in immunocompromised patients, resulting in our inability to demonstrate its efficacy, even when there appeared to be an appropriate anti-HBs response."

Rarely, there may be more to learn from an intervention's influence on the antecedent than on the endpoint itself! In a randomized trial among 6,024 patients with acute chest pain seen by paramedics outside of a hospital (Koster and Dunning, 1985), half were given an intramuscular injection of 400 mg of lidocaine; the other half were not. During the first hour following randomization, 8 treated patients developed ventricular fibrillation, in contrast to 17 in the control group. However, because prompt defibrillation was available, only 2 patients in each group with ventricular fibrillation died during the first hour; in-hospital mortality was also quite similar between the 2 groups. Although it is reasonable to conclude from these results that administration of lidocaine by defibrillator-equipped paramedics offers little or no reduction in cardiac mortality (the relevant endpoint in the population studied), in a population to whom out-of-hospital defibrillation is *not* available, greater attention should be given to the results for the antecedent condition, ventricular fibrillation. In such a population, the occurrence of out-of-hospital ventricular fibrillation would likely be strongly predictive of mortality.

Control of the Potentially Distorting Influence of Other Variables

The University Group Diabetes Project (UGDP) was a randomized trial of the ability of hypoglycemic agents to reduce the occurrence of complications of diabetes. One group of patients was assigned, at random, to receive the drug tolbutamide. These patients happened to differ from those who received no active agent in several respects (e.g., age) so that, apart from any influence of the drug, the tolbutamide therapy group would have been expected to have a somewhat higher rate of complications (Committee for the Assessment of Biometric Aspects of Controlled Trials of Hypoglycemic Agents, 1975).

This sort of imbalance can occur because, with respect to other relevant characteristics, randomization merely assures that *on the average* there will be equality of the groups being compared. In any one trial, between-group differences in characteristics related to the study outcome can occur (e.g., in the UGDP study), although in large trials only rarely are they of any appreciable magnitude.

Two strategies are commonly used to prevent the true measure of efficacy of a therapy from being distorted (confounded) in this way:

1. During the process of randomization, it is possible to form subgroups ("blocks") of subjects who are homogenous for the presence or level of risk factors for the study outcome and then to allocate a fixed proportion of the subjects within each block to each of the various treatments. For example, in the study of coronary artery bypass surgery (Principal Investigators of CASS and Associates, 1981), patients were put into groups based on their symptoms, ventricular function, number of diseased vessels, and the institution in which the treatment was being administered. Within each group, equal numbers were assigned to receive medical therapy and surgery, the order of the assignment being selected at random by the study's statisticians.

2. When the study has been concluded, the treatment groups can be compared for all characteristics believed to have an influence on the outcome. For those characteristics that differ among the groups, it will be possible to control analytically for their interfering effect, either through adjustment or through other statistical means (Rothman, 1977). In the UGDP study, for example, the difference in mortality from cardiovascular disease between subjects assigned to receive tolbutamide and those assigned to receive placebo—an excess of 13.2 per 1,000 per year in the tolbutamide treatment group—

was due in part to the higher mean age of the tolbutamide-treated group. The difference fell to 12.4 per 1,000 per year once the age distributions of the 2 groups were "forced" to be the same by an adjustment procedure.

When to Count Endpoints

Trials that tabulate the occurrence of certain *events* as the study endpoint(s)— for example, mortality, tumor recurrence, myocardial reinfarction, or rehospitalization —generally include all such events that occur among participants following randomization. However, to gain an understanding of the means by which an intervention may be effective, it can be useful to restrict the analysis of events to those that occur during particular times after the intervention has been administered.

Example: In the randomized trial of intramuscular lidocaine prophylaxis by paramedics for patients with suspected myocardial infarction (Koster and Dunning, 1985), the following data were obtained:

Occurrence of ventricular fibrillation after randomization	Lidocaine (n=2,987)	Control (n=3,037)
Within 0–15 minutes	6	5
Within 16–60 minutes	2	12
Total	8	17

The investigators argued that, because studies of lidocaine absorption following intramuscular injection suggested that blood levels in the first 15 minutes would be "subtherapeutic," particular attention should be given to a comparison of events occurring within 16–60 minutes. However, others (Gamble and Cohn, 1972; Geddes et al., 1974) who have speculated that low levels of lidocaine could actually predispose to ventricular fibrillation might argue that all events should be counted, irrespective of time since randomization. In practice, probably both comparisons should be presented. It is necessary to have one comparison in which no pharmacologic assumptions are made (i.e., the comparison of all instances of fibrillation). However, we should also allow for the possibility that our assumptions actually are correct and in a second analysis tailor our choice of the relevant time interval to match those assumptions.

Example: Recognition of the possibility that an intervention to lower serum cholesterol will provide a delayed benefit has led to long-term follow-up of participants in cholesterol-lowering trials. From a combined analysis of all such trials (Law et al., 1994), there is reason to believe that the measured impact of lowering cholesterol during the first several years after initiation of treatment may substantially underestimate the benefit in the years to follow.

For those trials that measure a patient's *status* as an endpoint (e.g., pain, mobility, physical exam, or laboratory findings), once the therapy has had sufficient time to exert its anticipated benefit it is somewhat arbitrary when the endpoint measurements are made. However, for recurring conditions in which therapy is being administered only transiently, it is necessary to assess outcome status both during and after therapy. For example, a study of the efficacy of a short-term (1–2 months) course of a benzodiazepine in the treatment of anxiety would need to monitor patients' psychological status not only while the drug was being taken but also after therapy had concluded. In the absence of the posttreatment assessment, the possibility of "rebound" following cessation—as has been observed in one randomized trial of a short course of a benzodiazepine (Power et al., 1985)—could not be considered.

Long-term measurement of status-type outcomes also is desirable if the effects of the intervention are likely to wane over time. A randomized trial of nicotine patches included an assessment of cigarette smoking not only in the short term (3 months) following administration of the patch (nicotine or placebo) but also at 1 year (Imperial Cancer Research Fund General Practice Research Group, 1994). The reason was that the investigators suspected, correctly, that in a number of patients smoking cessation would be maintained only transiently.

Handling Those Subjects Who Were Assigned to One Mode of Therapy but Who Did Not Receive It

Studies vary regarding the frequency with which participants, once randomized, fail to receive fully the treatment to which they have been assigned. It is the rare study in which the original assignments are adhered to perfectly. The reason for a change in therapy may be physician-initiated. Perhaps the condition of a patient assigned to the medical arm of a study of coronary artery surgery worsens, and the physician feels that surgery is necessary. Or perhaps a patient develops an adverse reaction to a study drug, and the physician must discontinue it. Alternatively, study participants themselves may decide to no longer adhere to the prescribed regimen.

The analysis of the results of a randomized trial should begin with a comparison of outcomes in groups of participants defined by their original treatment assignment, irrespective of the actual receipt of that treatment. This approach ("intention to treat") will retain the balance across groups, with respect to potential confounding factors, that randomization produces (Fisher et al., 1990). Categorizing patients on the basis of therapy received may introduce bias. That is, this strategy would permit the results to be distorted by the presence of one or more characteristics of persons who did not receive or complete the originally assigned therapy that also are correlated with the outcome being measured. Based on what we know about the reasons for changes in therapy following randomization and on characteristics and outcomes of patients who do change therapies, a considerable amount of bias would be expected to result in most studies. For instance, there are therapies that, if effective, are expected to produce demonstrable improvement in the patient's status before the full course of therapy is finished. If one form of treatment being evaluated truly is less effective, patients assigned to receive that treatment will less often experience demonstrable improvement, and thus they may be more likely not to complete the full course of therapy. In such situations, the exclusion of patients with an incomplete course of therapy from the analysis would diminish the measured efficacy of the superior therapy.

Even when the outcome does not influence compliance in such a direct way, the failure to maintain originally assigned groups can lead to a biased result. An instructive example comes from a study in which, in an effort to reduce cardiac mortality, the drug clofibrate (which lowers the concentration of serum cholesterol) or a placebo was prescribed to patients who had sustained a myocardial infarction (Coronary Drug Project Research Group, 1980). During the 5-year period of the study, adherence to the prescribed regimen was monitored in both treatment and placebo groups. The cumulative mortality was found not to differ between the clofibrate and placebo treatment groups. However, no matter which regimen had been prescribed, those who adhered to it 80% or more of the time experienced a cumulative mortality of about 15%, whereas the mortality in persons who were less compliant was about 27%. If, in the analysis, the investigators had placed the noncompliant clofibrate patients into the placebo group, they would have observed a spurious benefit associated with the use of the drug. A similar relation between nonadherence and increased mortality has been noted in a randomized trial of propanolol following myocardial infarction (Horwitz et al., 1990).

Example: There have been instances in which nonadherence among members of the control arm of a randomized trial has been frequent enough to diminish the value of the trial in identifying an impact of the intervention measure. This occurred in a study of hypertensive, moderately hypercholesterolemic patients who were randomly assigned either to receive 40 mg per day of pravastatin ($n = 5,170$) or to the "usual care" provided by their physicians ($n = 5,185$) (ALLHAT Officers and Coordinators for the ALLHAT Collaborative Research Group, 2002). The 6-year cumulative incidence of coronary disease events was 9.3% in the group assigned to receive pravastatin and 10.4% in the comparison group (relative risk = 0.91, 95% confidence interval = 0.79–1.04). However, during the trial approximately 30% of the comparison patients also began to take pravastatin or another lipid-lowering drug. Largely as a consequence of this, at year 4 of the trial the mean serum cholesterol levels had fallen in patients in both arms of the trial, by 17% in the pravastatin group and by 8% in the "usual care" group. Thus benefit of pravastatin treatment against the occurrence of coronary disease almost certainly exceeds that estimated in this trial. Such an inference is supported by an examination of the size of the relative risk across all studies of statin treatment, as a function of the difference in serum lipids between treatment and control arms that was achieved in each trial (Figure 4.3). The beneficial impact of statin therapy on risk of both the rate of all-cause mortality and the incidence of coronary heart disease (CHD) appears to grow in relation to the size of the differential reduction in lipid levels, with the study just described having the smallest differential reduction.

The disadvantage of retaining study participants in their originally assigned groups is that, in the presence of nonadherence to treatment assignment, the observed impact of therapy in outcomes across groups generally will be a diluted estimate of the true difference. If the level of nonadherence is very high, and if important predictors of outcome have been measured and can be controlled for, an analysis that ignores the randomization (and thus categorizes participants according to treatment received) might be the only hope of salvaging any useful information from the study.

More commonly when nonadherence is an issue, an intent-to-treat analysis is supplemented by one that attempts to deal with this problem in some manner that is less prone to bias than an analysis based simply on actual treatment received. For example, in a trial in which postmenopausal women were assigned to receive either combination estrogen-progestin therapy or placebo for approximately 5 years, one of the key outcomes was the incidence of venous thromboembolism (Cushman et al., 2004). The women assigned to receive hormone therapy experienced 2.1 times the risk of venous thromboembolism of women assigned to receive placebo. However, because about one-third of women in the hormone arm of the trial stopped taking the medication during the course of the study, and because a number of placebo recipients began to take hormones, the observed association is likely to be smaller than that which would have been observed in the absence of noncompliance. The investigators sought to deal with this problem by doing a supplemental analysis, one that included the experience of participants during the time they were adherent to their treatment assignment and, if they stopped being adherent, for 6 months thereafter. This analysis ignored outcome events and person-time that accrued in women beyond 6 months from the time they stopped taking their study medication. The results of the supplemental analysis suggested that current receipt of hormone therapy (or that which ended no more than 6 months earlier) increased a woman's risk of venous thromboembolism by a factor of 3.2, in contrast to the intent-to-treat estimate of 2.1.

If it could be assumed that the reason for discontinuation of the assigned regimen was unrelated to the incidence of venous thromboembolism, an even more accurate risk estimate would have resulted from restricting the analysis to just that period of time in which each participant was compliant. The investigators undoubtedly felt that such an assumption may not be valid but also that, whatever the basis for discontinuers being at altered risk of thromboembolism, altered risk would be present only transiently following

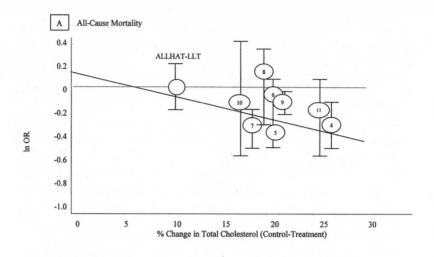

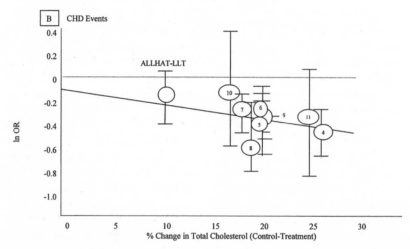

Figure 4.3 Reductions in mortality and coronary heart disease (CHD) event rates versus total serum cholesterol, randomized trials of cholesterol-lowering therapy. Log odds rations (ln OR) and 95% confidence intervals for active treatment versus control for 9 large statin trials are compared with regression lines (solid) from meta-analyses of 45 long-term trials using statins and other cholesterol-lowering interventions published before December 31, 2000. Numbers inside data markers are references. (Excerpted from the ALLHAT Officers and Coordinators, for the ALLHAT Collaborative Research Group, 2002.)

hormone discontinuation. In this instance, they made an educated guess that "transiently" might correspond to 6 months (after treatment cessation) and used this interval in their analysis.

In the preceding example, the focus was on the potential impact of an intervention (hormone therapy) during the time that it was being administered. If, instead, it is hypothesized that an intervention has an influence on the outcome in question even after that intervention has ended (e.g., prior hormone use and the incidence of breast cancer), then the analytic approach described previously to examine the incidence of venous thromboembolism would not be appropriate.

In the circumstance that the noncompliance cannot be a result of some untoward effect of the treatment—for example, when some persons enrolled in a trial never receive the intervention at all—steps can be taken to remove the bias associated with the inclusion of such persons in the analysis. This approach necessitates monitoring the occurrence of outcome events both in compliers and noncompliers.

Example: In a study conducted in rural Indonesia (Sommer and Zeger, 1991), 12,094 children in randomly selected villages were offered a large oral vitamin A supplement, and 11,588 children in other villages were not.

The following table summarizes the results for mortality in the 8 months following the time of the intervention in 11,588 control children, 9,675 children who actually received the supplement, and the other 2,419 children who were assigned to receive vitamin A but who did not.

Study group	Complied	# of children	Deaths	Mortality (per 1000)
Control	—	11,588	74	6.4
Vitamin A	—	12,094	46	3.8
	Yes	9,675	12	1.2
	No	2,419	34	14.1

The comparison of cumulative mortality in control children and all children offered vitamin A accurately assesses the relative *effectiveness* of the program (3.8 ÷ 6.4 = 0.59, or a 41% mortality reduction), as this incorporates the inability of the program to administer vitamin A to every child selected for supplementation. Yet the *efficacy* of the intervention is not as great as the ratio of rates between children who actually took the supplement and control children—1.2 ÷ 6.4 = 0.19, or an 81% mortality reduction—because those who took vitamin A had an inherently low risk of death. Note the atypically *high* cumulative mortality (14.1 per 1,000) in the children assigned to take vitamin A but who did not do so. In order to accurately estimate efficacy, it is first necessary to estimate the cumulative mortality in those control children who, if offered the supplement, would have taken it (x):

$$6.4 \text{ per } 1,000 = x \left(\frac{9675}{12094} \right) + 14.1 \text{ per } 1,000 \left(\frac{2419}{12,094} \right),$$

and $x = 4.47$ per 1,000.

Thus, based on these results, the relative risk associated with receipt of vitamin A supplementation is $1.24 \div 4.47 = 0.28$.

An elaboration of the preceding approach, one that allows for non-compliance in the control arm of the trial, has been provided by Cuzick et al (1997).

Evaluation of Treatment Efficacy in Subgroups of the Randomized Patient Population

Often a therapy will work for some patients but not for others. Perhaps, if the treatment is a drug, peculiarities of absorption or metabolism can render an otherwise useful drug ineffective in some patients. Or perhaps the "disease" we are treating is not a single entity and only some patients are capable of responding to the intervention we have chosen—consider the differential sensitivity of women with breast cancer to tamoxifen therapy depending on whether their tumors are estrogen-receptor positive or negative (Early Breast Cancer Trialists' Collaborative Group, 1992).

Recognizing that treatment efficacy can be modified by such characteristics of patients and/or their diseases, it is desirable to explore the results of a randomized controlled trial for the presence of subgroups of particularly sensitive or insensitive patients. Such an analysis can be done easily, given the original data, by making treatment-control comparisons in patients with and without a particular characteristic (e.g., a receptor-positive breast tumor) or in patients at 2 or more levels of a graded characteristic (e.g., levels of blood pressure).

Unfortunately, a difference between subgroups with regard to apparent treatment efficacy often cannot be so easily *interpreted*. We know that any given observed difference in outcome between treatment groups could be the result of chance alone; that is, it is not truly present in the "universe" of patients beyond the "sample" under study. The more subgroups we explore in our analysis, the greater the likelihood that, by chance, one or more will emerge in which the size of the treatment-control difference (or lack thereof) will differ from that of patients in general (Pocock and Hughes, 1990; Altman and Matthews, 1996).

With this in mind, when we see an apparent benefit of therapy restricted to (or enhanced in) a particular category of patient, it is prudent to remain skeptical. Occasionally, a very large intersubgroup difference that has a plausible explanation might be accepted as bona fide on the basis of a single study. If the expectation of a difference is strong enough, even a moderate degree of observed variation in response to treatment may be interpreted, tentatively, as evidence of a true difference.

> *Example:* Bracken et al. (1990) conducted a multicenter randomized trial in which a high dose of methylprednisolone or placebo was given to patients with acute spinal cord injury who were seen within 14 hours of their injuries. A difference between the treatment groups with regard to improvement in motor function 6 weeks and 6 months later was largely restricted to the approximately 50% of patients who received therapy within the first 8 hours after injury. Because the authors believed that the high dose of methylprednisolone was interfering with pathophysiologic processes that were present primarily in the first 8 hours following spinal cord injury, they felt justified in placing emphasis on the subgroup analysis in their publication and in concluding that "methylprednisolone in the dose used in this study improves neurologic recovery when the medication is given in the first eight hours."

Far more often, though, intergroup differences in outcome related to treatment observed in a single study need to be confirmed in other studies before therapeutic decisions would be affected.

Analysis and Reporting of Randomized Controlled Trials

The topic of statistical analysis of trials lies outside the scope of this book. An excellent introduction to the subject, one that emphasizes practical aspects and provides examples, can be found in an article by Peto et al. (1977).

Guidelines for reporting the results of randomized trials have been recommended (Moher et al., 2001) and are now commonly adhered to. These guidelines consist of a checklist of 22 items, as well as a flow diagram that summarizes recruitment into, and attrition from, the study.

When to Stop a Randomized Controlled Trial

The question as to when a randomized trial should be stopped has been examined in some detail by Pocock (1992). It is clear that the decision to continue such a trial involves at minimum a consideration of:

1. The size and direction of the observed difference between treatment groups;
2. The likelihood that chance could be responsible for the observed difference if a difference does not truly exist; and
3. The size of the difference between standard and new therapies that would be required for the latter to be more broadly introduced into clinical practice.

It is equally clear that the persons doing the considering should not be the study investigators but rather a group formed specifically for this purpose who can review the data and advise the investigators. The presence of an independent group can maximize the chances that the study results will adequately inform decision making for future patients, while not jeopardizing the right of study participants to receive the best "known" therapy.

Limitations of Randomized Controlled Trials

Randomized trials generally are not cheap to conduct. A considerable expenditure of resources is required to assemble a group of subjects, coordinate the administration of the randomization and treatment, and monitor the subjects over time. There are also substantial administrative costs associated with the multi-institutional collaboration that often is required. Because the magnitude of the cost is in part related to the number of subjects studied, there are usually financial restrictions on the size of most randomized trials.

Of course, the smaller the number of subjects, the smaller will be the ability of the trial to reliably determine the difference between treatment groups. The following example illustrates the ambiguities in interpretation that can arise when a seemingly large study is not quite large enough:

Example: Administration of zidovudine during the third trimester of pregnancy to a woman infected with HIV reduces the likelihood of transmission to her infant. To reduce that risk even further, a randomized trial was conducted in Thailand during the years 2001–2003 (Lallemant et al., 2004). HIV-positive women receiving zidovudine were assigned to receive a 200 mg oral dose of nevirapine or placebo during labor. Infants of mothers in the nevirapine group were further randomized to receive an oral suspension of nevirapine or placebo 2–3 days after birth. (All infants were formula fed and also were given zidovudine.)

An interim analysis of this study observed a much higher incidence of transmission in the absence of prenatal nevirapine treatment. This arm of the trial was stopped, and the study continued with a comparison only of infants who were and were not given nevirapine (among nevirapine-treated mothers). Of 705 infants given nevirapine, 212 (1.9%) were infected with HIV at 6 months of age, in contrast to 17 of 697 infants (2.8%) who received a placebo. The 95% confidence interval around the difference of 0.9 per 100 was –0.8, 2.6 per 100, that is, a single maternal dose of nevirapine was "statistically noninferior" to a maternal plus infant dose in blocking transmission of HIV.

In response to the findings of this trial, the ministry of public health in Thailand recommended nevirapine treatment for both an HIV-positive pregnant woman *and* (after delivery) her child. It is likely that the plausibility of there being a true benefit of nevirapine treatment of infants, combined with the treatment's relative safety and low cost, led the ministry to put aside concerns regarding the statistical uncertainty inherent in the trial's results. Whether the ministry's decision was wise or not, the point is that even in

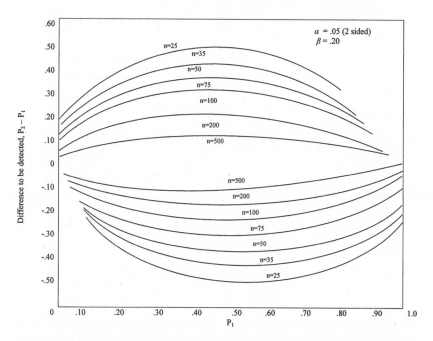

Figure 4.4 Sample sizes required for testing two independent proportions, P_1 and P_2, with 80% probability of obtaining a significant result at the 5% (two-sided) level. $n =$ number of observations *per group*. (Adapted from Feigel P. A graphical aid for determining sample size when comparing two independent proportions. Department of Biostatistics, Technical Report No. 6. Seattle: University of Washington; July 1977.)

a randomized trial in which some 1,400 participants were enrolled, chance remained a plausible explanation for a difference in the frequency of transmission (about 0.9 per 100) that, if genuine, would be of concern. *Differences in efficacy between treatment regimens that are of clinical importance often cannot be resolved in a randomized trial because of the trial's inability to enroll enough patients.*

Figure 4.4 depicts the number of subjects (n) needed in each of 2 groups of equal size to reliably (80% of the time) detect a statistically significant difference among them ($P < 0.05$). The number is related to (a) the frequency with which the study endpoint occurs in 1 of the groups (ρ_1, ranging from 0 to 1.0) and (b) the true difference between the frequency of the study endpoint in the 2 groups ($\rho_2 - \rho_1$), illustrated for values ranging from −0.5 to 0.6). So, for example, if 30% of patients with a given condition show symptomatic improvement after treatment with a placebo, and if in truth 50% treated with drug A improve ($\rho_2 - \rho_1 = 0.50 - 0.30 = 0.20$), then it will require slightly fewer than 200 patients (slightly fewer than 100 per group) to reliably identify this difference. Note that for between-group differences smaller than 0.10, several hundred or more patients per treatment group are needed. If there is but a small benefit from the therapy being evaluated, a large study is required to document that benefit.

Questions

4.1. The following is paraphrased from an article published several years ago on the evaluation of the efficacy of a group of drugs:

> We do not discuss randomized controlled trials of these drugs because our concern has been to evaluate the effects of the drugs on populations rather than on individuals. Thus, although randomized controlled trials provide unique information on the effects of drugs, they would concern us only if the study groups were representative of defined subgroups of the general population. Such representation is rarely possible in these trials, which generally involve volunteers.

You disagree with the opinion expressed here. Why?

4.2. Luesley et al. (1988) conducted a randomized controlled trial to assess the efficacy of subsequent therapy in women with advanced ovarian cancer who had undergone primary laparotomy and an attempt to resect as much tumor as possible. In a portion of the study, 2 treatment groups were formed following the patients' recovery from surgery: (a) cisplatin, 5 doses of 100 mg/m^2, followed by 12 two-week courses of chlorambucil (0.2 mg/kg/day); and (b) cisplatin and chlorambucil as in (a), except that following the cisplatin therapy a second-look laparatomy was to be done, during which an attempt would be made to remove additional malignant tissue.

Unfortunately, the planned treatment could not be carried out in all patients. Of 53 women assigned to group (b), 21 did not receive second-look surgery after all, either because of clinically evident progressive disease or because the patient changed her mind about undergoing surgery. During the follow-up period (median of 46 months for both groups), 44 of 57 women (77%) in group (a) died, in comparison to 42 of 53 women (79%) in group (b).

Aside from increasing the number of subjects, what alteration in the design of this study would have contributed most to increasing its ability to detect a true beneficial effect of second-look laparotomy, as a complement to treatment with cisplatin and chlorambucil, on survival in women with advanced ovarian cancer?

4.3. A program of semiannual screening for asymptomatic bacteriuria led to the identification of 358 elderly women with urinary tract infection (Abrutyn et al., 1994). These women were assigned at random to receive either a short course (1–3 days) of an antibiotic to which the infecting organism was believed to be sensitive or a placebo. Women positive on reculture 5–10 days later were treated either for 14 additional days with an antibiotic appropriate for the bacterium that was found or for 14 additional days with placebo.

Short-term eradication of bacteriuria occurred in 82.9% of women who received antibiotic therapy, but in only 15.6% of those given placebo. Over a period of up to 9 years, 18.1% of the antibiotic-treated women died, versus 20.3% of the control women (relative rate = 0.9, 95% confidence interval = 0.5–1.5). Nonfatal outcomes were not assessed.

The authors concluded, "Within the limitations of this study, our results provide evidence that asymptomatic bacteriuria in the elderly should not be treated if the goal is to decrease mortality." What is the primary limitation of this study that prevents you from concluding that antibiotic treatment of an elderly woman with an asymptomatic urinary tract infection would not result in some decrease in her risk of death?

4.4. Antiepileptic drugs can have a detrimental effect on cognitive function and behavior. Thus a randomized trial was done to determine the consequences of gradual withdrawal of these drugs in persons who had been taking them for at least 2 years and had been seizure-free during that time (Medical Research Council Antiepileptic Drug Withdrawal Study Group, 1991). In the 2-year period following randomization, seizures recurred in 41% of patients whose medication had been discontinued, but in only 22% of those continued on antiepileptic therapy.

No placebo was used in this trial because (among other reasons given) "placebo substitution is not a clinical option in the management of patients in remission [from seizures]." Is this a compelling rationale?

4.5. In the late 1990s, a randomized controlled trial of the efficacy of screening for abdominal aortic aneurysm was conducted in Perth, Australia (Norman et al., 2004). Male residents of the city ages 65–83 years were assigned either to be or not to be invited to attend an ultrasound exam, with results of the exam provided to the patient and his general practitioner for further action (e.g., surgical referral or follow-up examination), if appropriate. The 2 groups were compared with respect to the occurrence of death from abdominal aortic aneurysm or its treatment following screening (or, among men in the control arm, the date they would have been screened had they been in the intervention arm). The results were as follows:

Intervention group	# of men	# of deaths*	Age-adjusted mortality**
Invited for screening	19,352	18	11.51
Attended	12,203	7	7.48
Did not attend	7,149	11	18.27
Not invited	19,352	25	18.91

*Deaths due to abdominal aortic aneurysm or its treatment
**Deaths per 100,000 man-years

Based on an intent-to-screen analysis, the mortality ratio (invited:not invited) was 11.51/18.91 = 0.61, with a 95% confidence interval of 0.33–1.11. The authors concluded that "screening for abdominal aortic aneurysm was not effective in men aged 65–83 years."

(a) How would you analyze the results of this trial to obtain a valid estimate of the efficacy of screening, one that is not distorted by the large proportion of invited men who declined to be screened?

(b) Based on that analysis, what is your estimate of the relative mortality (from abdominal aortic aneurysm or its treatment) associated with receipt of abdominal ultrasound screening in this population?

Answers

4.1. Randomized controlled trials almost always involve volunteers, so there will almost always be a need to generalize to a reference population that is not entirely similar to the study population; the former will contain potential nonvolunteers as well. The alternative approaches to evaluating drug efficacy, however—one of the nonrandomized designs—have a potentially more important drawback: Patients who receive and do not receive the drug are likely to have inherently different risks of the outcome that the therapy seeks to prevent.

So, in our search for internally valid studies, we pay particular attention to the results of randomized controlled trials, and we certainly do not eschew them. The process of generalizing to a reference population may still be tricky, but it cannot even begin until there is confidence that the comparison among the study subjects themselves has some validity.

4.2. The randomization of patients should have been performed following, rather than prior to, the administration of the initial chemotherapy (cisplatin). In that way, women with clinically evident metastatic disease—who are not candidates for second-look surgery—could have been excluded from both groups (b) and (a). So, too, could women who were unwilling to undergo reoperation at that time. The inclusion of all these women in the group to be randomized, which necessitates their inclusion in the analysis, guarantees a diluted estimate of any true benefit associated with second-look surgery.

4.3. Even if eradication of asymptomatic urinary tract infections in elderly women truly leads to a reduced death rate from some causes (e.g., from chronic renal disease), it is unlikely that these causes would constitute more than a small proportion of the total mortality experience. Thus the study's finding of an 11% reduction in mortality among antibiotic-treated women (20.3% – 18.1%/20.3%)—a result that could easily have occurred by chance given no true influence of antibiotic treatment of asymptomatic urinary infections on mortality—may well be the largest true reduction that plausibly could have occurred. In order for a randomized trial to contribute in a meaningful way to the decision to screen for and/or treat asymptomatic bacteriuria in the elderly, that trial must: (a) be *much* larger than the one conducted and/or (b) examine endpoints (e.g., death from kidney disease, development of renal dysfunction or urinary symptoms) whose occurrence would be affected to a relatively greater degree than would total mortality.

4.4. Placebo substitution is rarely if ever a clinical option in the management of any condition. Thus, if this rationale put forth by the authors were sound, there would be no randomized trials in which a placebo was used! A placebo is incorporated into the design of a randomized trial only because blinding of study participants and study personnel maximizes the likelihood of the trial producing a valid result.

In the study of seizure recurrence in relation to drug withdrawal, it is conceivable that some of the difference observed is due to differences in seizure reporting that resulted from the lack of blinding. However, the fact that there was a difference in the reported incidence of tonic-clonic seizures—the most severe form and the one least susceptible to differential completeness of reporting—argues that not all of the difference could be due to this potential source of bias.

4.5. In this study, the ability to estimate the efficacy of screening by means of a direct comparison of the mortality experience of the originally randomized groups has been seriously compromised by the high proportion of invited men who were not screened ($7,149/19,352 = 36.9\%$). However, because: (a) noncompliance could not have been a consequence of the attempted intervention and (b) deaths have been ascertained in all men invited for screening (whether or not they attended), it is possible to use the data gathered in the trial to obtain an unbiased estimate of the efficacy of screening for abdominal aortic aneurysm. One does this by comparing the rate of death from abdominal aortic aneurysm and its treatment between the screened group and that portion of the not-invited group who, had they been invited, *would* have attended (see p. 70). In this instance, the latter rate is estimated to be

$$\frac{18.91 \text{ per } 100,000 - 18.27 \text{ per } 100,000 \ (0.369)}{0.631} = 19.28 \text{ per } 100,000 \text{ man-years}$$

Therefore, the relative mortality from abdominal aortic aneurysm and its treatment among screened men is estimated to be

$$(7.48 \text{ per } 100,000) / (19.28 \text{ per } 100,000) = 0.39,$$

a much different value than the relative mortality of 0.61 calculated in the intent-to-treat analysis.

References

Abrutyn E, Mossey J, Berlin JA, et al. Does asymptomatic bacteriuria predict mortality and does antimicrobial treatment reduce mortality in elderly ambulatory women? *Ann Intern Med* 1994;120:827–833.

Adachi JD, Bensen WG, Brown J, et al. Intermittent etidronate therapy to prevent corticosteroid-induced osteoporosis. *New Engl J Med* 1997;337:382–387.

ALLHAT Officers and Coordinators for the ALLHAT Collaborative Research Group. Major outcomes in moderately hypercholesterolemic, hypertensive patients randomized to pravastatin vs usual care. *JAMA* 2002;288:2998–3007.

Altman DG, Matthews JNS. Interaction 1: Heterogeneity of effect. *Br Med J* 1996;313:486.

Aspirin Myocardial Infarction Study Research Group. A randomized controlled trial of aspirin in persons recovered from myocardial infarction. *JAMA* 1980;243:661–669.

Australian National Health and Medical Research Council Dietary Salt Study Management Committee. Fall in blood pressure with modest reduction in salt intake in mild hypertension. *Lancet* 1989;1:399–402.

Bracken MB, Shepard MJ, Collins WF, et al. A randomized, controlled trial of methylprednisolone or naloxone in the treatment of acute spinal-cord injury. *N Engl J Med* 1990;322:1405–1411.

Buchwald H, Vargo RL, Matts JP, et al. Effect of partial ileal bypass surgery on mortality and morbidity from coronary heart disease in patients with hypercholesterolemia. *N Engl J Med* 1990;323:946–955.

Byar DP, Herzberg AM, Tan WY. Incomplete factorial designs for randomized clinical trials. *Stat Med* 1993;12:1629–1641.

Carette S, LeClaire R, Marcoux S, et al. Epidural corticosteroid injections for sciatica due to herniated nucleus pulposus. *New Engl J Med* 1997;336:1634–1640.

Church TR, Elerer F, Mandel JS. RE: All-cause mortality in randomized trials of cancer screening. *J Natl Cancer Inst* 2002;94:861.

Cobb LA, Thomas GI, Dillard DH, et al. An evaluation of internal-mammary artery ligation by a double-blind technic. *N Engl J Med* 1959;260:1115–1118.

Committee for the Assessment of Biometric Aspects of Controlled Trials of Hypoglycemic Agents. Report of the committee for the assessment of biometric aspects of controlled trials of hypoglycemic agents. *JAMA* 1975;231:583–608.

Committee of Principal Investigators. A co-operative trial in the primary prevention of ischemic heart disease using clofibrate. *Br Heart J* 1978;40:1069–1118.

Coope J, Thompson JM, Poller I. Effects of "natural estrogen" replacement therapy on menopausal symptoms and blood clotting. *Br Med J* 1975;4:139–143.

Coronary Drug Project Research Group. Aspirin in coronary heart disease. *J Chron Dis* 1976;29:625–642.

Coronary Drug Project Research Group. Influence of adherence to treatment and response of cholesterol on mortality in the coronary drug project. *N Engl J Med* 1980;303:1038–1041.

Cushman M, Kuller LH, Prentice R, et al. Estrogen plus progestin and risk of venous thrombosis. *JAMA* 2004;292:1573–1580.

Cuzick J, Edwards R, Segnan N. Adjusting for non-compliance and contamination in randomized clinical trials. *Statistics in Medicine* 1997;16:1017–1029.

Dayton S, Pearce MI, Hashimoto S, et al. A controlled clinical trial of a diet high in unsaturated fat in preventing complications of atherosclerosis. *Circulation* 1969;39–40 (suppl 2):1–63.

Diabetic Retinopathy Study Research Group. Photocoagulation treatment of proliferative diabetic retinopathy: Clinical application of diabetic retinopathy study (DRS) findings. DRS Report Number 8. *Ophthalmology* 1981; 88:583–600.

Early Breast Cancer Trialists' Collaborative Group. Systemic treatment of early breast cancer by hormonal, cytotoxic, or immune therapy. *Lancet* 1992;339:1–15.

Echt DS, Liebson PR, Mitchell LB, et al. Mortality and morbidity in patients receiving encainide, flecainide, or placebo. *N Engl J Med* 1991;324:781–788.

Ellenberg SS. Randomization designs in comparative clinical trials. *N Engl J Med* 1984;310:1404–1408.

Ellenberg SS, Temple R. Placebo-controlled trials and active-control trials in the evaluation of new treatments. *Ann Intern Med* 2000;133:464–470.

Emanuel EJ, Miller FG. The ethics of placebo-controlled trials: A middle ground. *N Engl J Med* 2001;345:915–918.

Fisher LD, Dixon DO, Herson J, et al. Intention to treat in clinical trials. In Peace KE (ed), *Statistical Issues in Drug Research and Development.* New York: Marcel Dekker, 1990.

Freedman B: Equipoise and the ethics of clinical research. *N Engl J Med* 1987;317:141–145.

Freemantle N, Calvert M, Wood, J, et al. Composite outcomes in randomized trials; greater precision but with greater uncertainty? *JAMA* 2003;289: 2554–2559.

Gamble OW, Cohn K. Effect of propanolol, procainamide, and lidocaine on ventricular automaticity and reentry in experimental myocardial infarction. *Circulation* 1972;46:498–596.

Geddes JS, Webb SW, Adgey AAJ. Effects of lidocaine on "gating" mechanism. *Am Heart J* 1974;88:260–261.

Gilchrest BA, Rowe JW, Brown RS, et al. Ultraviolet phototherapy of uremic pruritus: Long-term results and possible mechanism of action. *Ann Intern Med* 1979;91:17–21.

Guyatt G, Sackett D, Taylor DW, et al. Determining optimal therapy—randomized trials in individual patients. *N Engl J Med* 1986;314:889–892.

Hills M, Armitage P. The two-period cross-over clinical trial. *Br J Clin Pharmacol* 1979;8:7–20.

Horwitz RI, Viscoli CM, Berkman L, et al. Treatment adherence and risk of death after a myocardial infarction. *Lancet* 1990;336:542–545.

Hypertension Detection and Follow-up Program Cooperative Group. Five-year findings of the Hypertension Detection and Follow-up Program: 1. Reduction in mortality of persons with high blood pressure, including mild hypertension. *JAMA* 1979a;242:2562–2571.

Hypertension Detection and Follow-up Program Cooperative Group. Five-year findings of the Hypertension Detection and Follow-up Program: 2. Mortality by race, sex, and age. *JAMA* 1979b;242:2572–2577.

Imperial Cancer Research Fund General Practice Research Group. Randomized trial of nicotine patches in general practice: Results at one year. *Br Med J* 1994;308:1476–1477.

Jain RK. Physiological barriers to delivery of monoclonal antibodies and other macromolecules in tumors. *Cancer Res* 1990;50:2741–2751.

Jones B, Jarvis P, Lewis JA, et al. Trials to assess equivalence: The importance of rigorous methods. *Br Med J* 1996;313:36–39.

Karlowski TR, Chalmers TC, Frenkel LD, et al. Ascorbic acid for the common cold: A prophylactic and therapeutic trial. *JAMA* 1975;231:1038–1042.

Koster RQ, Dunning AJ. Intramuscular lidocaine for prevention of lethal arrhythmias in the prehospitalization phase of acute myocardial infarction. *N Engl J Med* 1985;313:1105–1110.

Kronmal RA, Cain KC, Ye Z, et al. Total serum cholesterol levels and mortality risk as a function of age: A report based on the Framingham data. *Arch Intern Med* 1993;152:1065–1073.

Lallemant M, Jourdain G, LeCoeur S, et al. Single-dose perinatal nevirapine plus standard zidovudine to prevent mother-to-child transmission of HIV-1 in Thailand. *N Engl J Med* 2004;351:217–228.

Last JM. *A Dictionary of Epidemiology.* 3rd ed. New York: Oxford, 1995.

Law MR, Wald NJ, Thompson SG. By how much and how quickly does reduction in serum cholesterol concentration lower risk of ischaemic heart disease? *Br Med J* 1994;308:367–373.

Lindor KD, for the Mayo Primary Sclerosing Cholangitis-Ursodeoxycholic Acid Study Group. Ursodial for primary sclerosing cholangitis. *N Engl J Med* 1997;336:691–695.

Lipid Research Clinics Program. The Lipid Research Clinics coronary primary prevention trial results. *JAMA* 1984;251:351–364.

Long-Term Intervention with Pravastatin in Ischaemic Disease (LIPID) Study Group. Prevention of cardiovascular events and death with pravastatin in patients with coronary heart disease and a broad range of initial cholesterol levels. *N Engl J Med* 1998;339:1349–1357.

Lorenz RI, Weber M, Kotzur J, et al. Improved aortocoronary bypass patency by low-dose aspirin (100 mg daily): Effects on platelet aggregation and thromboxane formation. *Lancet* 1984;1:1261–1264.

Louis TA, Lavori PW, Bailar JC, et al. Crossover and self-controlled designs in clinical research. *N Engl J Med* 1984;310:24–31.

Lubsen J, Pocock SJ. Factorial trials in cardiology: Pros and cons. *Eur Heart J* 1994;15:585–588.

Luesley D, Blackledge G, Kelly K, et al. Failure of second-look laparotomy to influence survival in epithelial ovarian cancer. *Lancet* 1988;2:599–603.

Margolin A, Kleber H, Avants SK, et al. Acupuncture for the treatment of cocaine addition. *JAMA* 2002;287:55–63.

McLeod RS, Cohen Z, Taylor DW, et al. Single-patient randomized clinical trial. *Lancet* 1986;1:726–728.

Medical Research Council Antiepileptic Drug Withdrawal Study Group. Randomised study of antiepileptic drug withdrawal in patients in remission. *Lancet* 1991;337:1175–1180.

Moher D, Schulz KF, Altman D for the CONSORT Group. The CONSORT Statement: Revised recommendations for improving the quality of reports of parallel-group randomized trials. *JAMA* 2001;285:1987–1991.

Norman PE, Jamrozik K, Lawrence-Brown MM, et al. Population based randomised controlled trial on impact of screening on mortality from abdominal aortic aneurysm. *Br Med J* 2004;329:1259–1262.

Peto R, Pike MC, Armitage NE, et al. Design and analysis of randomized clinical trials requiring prolonged observation of each patient: 2. Analysis and examples. *Br J Cancer* 1977;35:1–39.

Pocock SJ. When to stop a clinical trial. *Br Med J* 1992;305:235–240.

Pocock SJ, Hughes MD. Estimation issues in clinical trials and overviews. *Stat Med* 1990;9:657–671.

Power KG, Jerron DWA, Rimpson RJ, et al. Controlled study of withdrawal symptoms and rebound anxiety after six week course of diazepam for generalized anxiety. *Br Med J* 1985;290:1246–1248.

Principal Investigators of CASS and Associates. The National Heart, Lung, and Blood Institute coronary artery surgery study. *Circulation* 1981;63 (suppl 1):11–181.

Riethmuller G, Schneider-Gadicke E, Schlimok G. Randomized trial of monoclonal antibody for adjuvant therapy of resected Dukes' C colorectal carcinoma. *Lancet* 1994;343:1177–1183.

Riggs BL, Hodgson SF, O'Fallon WM. Effects of fluoride treatment on the fracture rate in postmenopausal women with osteoporosis. *N Engl J Med* 1990;322:802–809.

Rosenberger WF, Lachin JM. *Randomization in Clinical Trials: Theory and Practice.* New York: John Wiley & Sons, 2002.

Rothman KJ. Epidemiologic methods in clinical trials. *Cancer* 1977;39(suppl 4):1771–1775.

Shapiro S, Strax P, Venet L. Periodic breast cancer screening in reducing mortality from breast cancer. *JAMA* 1971;215:1777–1785.

Shepherd J, Blauw GJ, Murphy MB, et al. Pravastatin in elderly individuals at risk of vascular disease (PROSPER): A randomised controlled trial. *Lancet* 2002;360:1623–1630.

Siscovick DS, Raghunathan TE, Psaty BM, et al. Diastolic blood pressure and the risk of primary cardiac arrest among pharmacologically-treated hypertensive patients. *J Gen Int Med* 1996;11:350–356.

Sommer A, Zeger SL. On estimating efficacy from clinical trials. *Statistics in Medicine* 1991;10:45–52.

Stein CM, Pincus T. Placebo-controlled studies in rheumatoid arthritis: Ethical issues. *Lancet* 1999;353:400–403.

Stenestrand U, Wallentin L for the Swedish Register of Cardiac Intensive Care (RIKS-HIA). Early statin treatment following acute myocardial infarction and 1-year survival. *JAMA* 2001;285:430–436.

Stevens CE, Alter HJ, Taylor PE, et al. Hepatitis B vaccine in patients receiving hemodialysis: Immunogenicity and efficacy. *N Engl J Med* 1984;311:496–500.

Storm T, Thamsborg G, Steiniches T, et al. Effect of intermittent cyclical etidronate therapy on bone mass and fracture rate in women with post-menopausal osteoporosis. *N Engl J Med* 1990;322:1265–1271.

Temple R, Ellenberg SS. Placebo-controlled trials and active-control trials in the evaluation of new treatments. *Ann Intern Med* 2000;133:455–463.

Veterans Administration Cooperative Study Group on Antihypertensive Agents. Effects of treatment on morbidity in hypertension: Results in patients with diastolic blood pressures averaging 115 through 129 mm Hg. *JAMA* 1967;212:116–122.

Watts NB, Harris ST, Genant HK, et al. Intermittent cyclical etidronate treatment of postmenopausal osteoporosis. *N Engl J Med* 1990;323:73–79.

Weiss NS, Koepsell TD. Re: All-cause mortality in randomized trials of cancer screening. *J Natl Cancer Inst* 2002;94:864–865.

Zelen M. A new design for randomized clinical trials. *N Engl J Med* 1979;300: 1242–1245.

Zelen M. Randomized consent designs for clinical trials: An update. *Stat Med* 1990;9:645–656.

5

Therapeutic Efficacy

Nonrandomized Studies

A randomized controlled trial is the best method of evaluating the efficacy of therapy. Nonetheless, therapeutic decisions often have to be made in the absence of results obtained in this way. Some therapeutic measures were introduced years ago, at a time when randomized trials were the exception rather than the rule. Other therapeutic measures, even today, often do not undergo evaluation in a randomized trial prior to being widely adopted: for instance, a dietary or environmental manipulation. Or perhaps a treatment has been tested and found to be modestly effective in a randomized controlled trial, but because the outcome under study was an intermediate one (e.g., control of high blood pressure in a trial of an antihypertensive agent), the influence of the treatment on the clinically relevant outcome (e.g., morbidity and mortality from cardiovascular disease) is uncertain. Finally, the results of a randomized trial utilizing the clinically relevant outcome may be suggestive of therapeutic efficacy, but because of the small size of the trial, the role of chance in generating these results cannot be statistically excluded (see Chapter 4).

In the absence of decisive data from one or more randomized trials, where can we turn for evidence that will make our therapeutic decision a more rational one? We must make an attempt to exploit the fact that, among patients with the same illness, it is often possible to find groups that happen to be treated in different ways. To evaluate the efficacy of the treatments relative to one another, the experiences of these patient groups following treatment are compared.

When Can We Trust Nonrandomized Studies to Provide a Valid Result?

Unfortunately, simple comparisons of groups of patients treated in different ways may be misleading, for the distribution of illness severity may not be similar among the groups. Patients with a mild form of an illness can receive one type of treatment, whereas persons with a more severe form can receive another. Thus the measured differences between the experiences of patient groups receiving alternative therapies may be attributable more to differences in characteristics of the patients themselves than to differences in the efficacy of the therapies. This is often termed "confounding by indication." For example, a comparison of the survival experience of persons with lung cancer who received (a) surgery followed by radiation therapy or (b) surgery alone would probably be biased in favor of the latter group, as supplemental radiation therapy is usually prescribed only for patients with demonstrable metastases, a sign of a particularly poor prognosis. Similarly, several series of patients with cirrhosis of the liver and esophageal varices who underwent shunt surgery had a better survival experience than did other cirrhotic patients with varices, but this difference now seems to have been due almost entirely to the poorer condition of the members of the nonsurgical group (Sacks et al., 1982).

Furthermore, among patients with a given illness there may be some who have other health problems that proscribe the use of one of several available therapies. For example, patients with end-stage renal disease who receive dialysis therapy have higher levels of comorbidity than those who receive cadaveric transplantation (Vollmer et al., 1983). Thus a simple comparison of survival in persons receiving these 2 modes of therapy would spuriously favor the transplant group.

Under what circumstances can data gathered outside randomized controlled trials be used to draw valid inferences concerning the efficacy of therapy? Not everyone offers the same answer to this question. Some say that results from studies in which randomization has not taken place can almost never be trusted, that the factors influencing the selection of certain patients for certain therapies are too strong to be overcome (Sacks et al., 1982; Pocock and Elbourne, 2000). However, based on their review of the literature, Benson and Hartz (2000) concluded that the "misuse of observational [i.e., nonrandomized] studies does not often occur" and that "our results suggest that observational studies usually do provide valid information." It does seem that, because we commonly employ the findings of nonrandomized studies to judge what might be done to prevent disease or to prevent adverse effects of therapy, these findings could play at least *some* role in allowing us to judge the benefits of therapy. For example, there are virtually no data from randomized controlled trials that have contributed to our conclusions that lung cancer could be prevented by not smoking cigarettes or that vaginal adenocarcinoma could be prevented by avoiding prenatal exposure to diethylstilbestrol (DES). On the other hand, the possibility for bias in using nonrandomized data to judge therapeutic efficacy is great, so it is particularly important to specify the conditions that must prevail in these studies so that the inferences drawn regarding efficacy can be valid.

At a minimum, a valid comparison between 2 or more treatment groups requires monitoring the course of the illness under treatment similarly among the groups. Whether the tools for monitoring are questionnaires, laboratory values, or medical or death records, the same tools must be applied in the same way for all subjects in order for the study's findings to be credible.

A second criterion for validity, sometimes more difficult to achieve than the one just mentioned, requires that at least 1 of 2 conditions must hold: (a) The size of the observed difference in outcome among the treatment groups substantially exceeds that which could be expected on the basis of plausible (but unmeasured) differences among the groups with respect to other characteristics that influence the outcome of illness (e.g., illness severity); (b) the differences among the various treatment groups, with respect to other factors that influence the outcome of illness, can be made sufficiently small (by means of appropriately matching subjects in the groups and/or making adjustments in the analysis) so as not to interfere with the evaluation of the influence of treatment per se.

Here are some examples in which condition (a) appears to have been met.

Example: A group of physicians performed bone marrow transplantation in 24 children who had relapsed after an initial course of chemotherapy for acute lymphoblastic leukemia (Johnson et al., 1981). At the end of a mean follow-up period of about 2 years, 11 children were alive (9 in remission), in contrast to only 2 of 21 (1 in remission) children who had relapsed but received only additional chemotherapy. The children had not been randomly assigned to the 2 treatment groups; rather, those who had an HLA-identical donor available were offered marrow transplantation; the others were not. A number of similarly designed nonrandomized evaluations of marrow transplantation for this indication have since been conducted (Boulad et al., 1999), with results similar to those of Johnson et al. (1981). There is no reason to believe that the availability of an HLA-identical donor correlates much, if at all, with survival in acute lymphoblastic leukemia. Thus it is very likely that the difference in survival is largely the difference in the efficacy of the 2 therapeutic approaches.

Example: Monson et al. (1973) followed 353 women treated for Stage I endometrial cancer at a single Boston hospital. Those who received radiation therapy after hysterectomy had a significantly greater 5-year survival than did those who had hysterectomy only. The fact that this difference occurred despite an initially poorer life expectancy (on the basis of tumor grade) in the irradiated group argues strongly for the efficacy of posthysterectomy irradiation in this condition. Randomized controlled trials of radiation therapy for high-grade endometrial cancer were conducted subsequently (and reviewed by Naumann [2002]).

They suggest a reduction in the rate of tumor recurrence and (to a lesser extent) mortality associated with receipt of radiation therapy and thus support the validity of an inference of efficacy from the results of the original nonrandomized study.

Example: In 1979, prior to the identification of the human immunodeficiency virus (HIV), some hemophilia centers began to use factor VIII concentrate that had been pasteurized at 60§C for 10 hours (Schimpf et al., 1989). This procedure, designed to rid the concentrate of hepatitis viruses, produced relatively low yields of factor VIII, not enough for all patients served by the centers. To determine whether this method of preparing the concentrate reduced the risk of transmission of HIV, 155 newly treated patients during the years1979–1986 who received it exclusively were checked for HIV antibodies after a mean follow-up of nearly 6 years. None was positive, whereas approximately 60% would have been expected to be, based on the experience of patients treated with unheated factor VIII concentrate.

Despite the absence of randomization, the large difference between the observed and expected frequency of HIV infection provides convincing evidence of the efficacy of pasteurization of factor VIII concentrate, especially because (a) the dose of factor VIII was not appreciably different between patients who received heated and unheated concentrate and because (b) it is hard to imagine that the reasons for selecting patients to receive the heated concentrate—its availability and the patients' apparent freedom from clinical hepatitis infection—could on their own have been responsible for all 155 patients being able to resist the development of HIV infection.

Example: For a woman with one of a number of germ-line BRCA1 or BRCA2 mutations, bilateral salpingo-oophorectomy offers the potential to reduce her subsequent incidence of ovarian cancer (although she may still develop a malignancy of the same cell lineage, papillary serous peritoneal carcinoma). No randomized trials have been conducted to document whether this potential benefit is realized. Two cohort studies (Kauff et al., 2002; Rebbeck et al., 2002) compared cancer incidence between women with these mutations who underwent the prophylactic surgery and those who chose not to do so. Whereas the 2 groups were comparable with regard to other potential risk factors for ovarian cancer (such as age and a history of not using oral contraceptives), the subsequent incidence of the combination of ovarian carcinoma/papillary serous peritoneal carcinoma differed by about a factor of 10 (higher in women who had not had prophylactic surgery). This large disparity, combined with the plausibility of the result and the *im*plausibility of any noncausal basis for it, argues strongly that prophylactic salpingo-oophorectomy in BRCA1 and BRCA2 mutation carriers offers considerable protection against the development of ovarian/peritoneal cancer.

Other investigators have started with treatment groups of inherently different prognoses, but, by identifying important prognostic characteristics and by matching or adjusting for them, they were able to achieve a fair degree of between-group comparability (i.e., their studies met the second condition for validity).

Example: To evaluate the efficacy of lidocaine prophylaxis in preventing death following acute myocardial infarction, the outcome of patients hospitalized with a myocardial infarction was monitored (Horwitz and Feinstein, 1981). In comparing the survival of patients who did and did not receive lidocaine prophylaxis, the investigators noted that some patients had ventricular tachycardia or other ventricular ectopic activity, conditions that mandated the use of lidocaine. Because these abnormalities are strongly predictive of mortality, inclusion of these patients in the analysis would bias the study toward finding a deleterious effect of lidocaine. Accordingly, the investigators chose to eliminate patients with ventricular tachycardia or other ventricular ectopic activity from their analysis. They also matched the groups being compared on other factors less strongly related to the risk of mortality—age, sex, race, and date of hospitalization.

Example: Psaty et al. (1991) investigated the efficacy of various treatments for high blood pressure in reducing the rate of myocardial infarction. Because the study was not randomized, there was concern that the results might be subject to confounding by indication, in that one class of antihypertensives—beta blockers—was also used in the treatment of coronary disease and its symptoms. With this in mind, 2 features were incorporated into the comparison of type of antihypertensive used in the several weeks prior to a heart attack by hypertensive patients and prior to a corresponding point in time by hypertensive controls: (a) patients with a prior diagnosis of coronary heart disease were excluded from the analysis; and (b) because onset of angina-like symptoms in the prior month (but not an onset earlier than that) was observed to be related to the risk of myocardial infarction, patients who began taking a particular antihypertensive agent during the prior month were excluded as well.

Example: In designing a study to evaluate the efficacy of a vaccine against pneumococcal pneumonia, investigators at the Centers for Disease Control and Prevention were confronted with the problem that many of those to whom the vaccine was being given—such as persons of advanced age or those with an immune disorder—were at far higher risk of contracting the disease than were other persons. Thus a simple comparison of disease rates in vaccinated and unvaccinated persons would be likely to seriously underestimate the efficacy of the vaccine. (A randomized controlled trial to evaluate this issue could be logistically difficult and extremely expensive to conduct. The recruitment of potential subjects, their follow-up for the occurrence of pneumonia, and the low rate of the disease are obstacles that have discouraged the conduct of such studies in high-risk individuals.) To deal with this problem, the investigators (Broome et al., 1980) took advantage of the fact that there are a number of types of *P. pneumoniae* and that the vaccine is directed at only a minority of them. So, among persons with pneumococcal pneumonia, they separated those in whom vaccine-type organisms were cultured from persons with other types of *P. pneumoniae*. Because there was no reason to believe that the 2 groups were different in their underlying risk of contracting pneumococcal pneumonia, a comparison of vaccination histories between the groups could be expected to provide a valid estimate of efficacy.

Example: Patients undergoing coronary bypass procedures involving the anterior descending artery typically receive either a vein graft or an internal mammary artery graft. To assess the long-term consequences of this choice, the survival of 3,625 vein graft and 2,306 internal mammary artery recipients during the 1970s was compared (Loop et al., 1986). The former group of patients had a slightly greater prevalence of multivessel disease and impaired left ventricular function, but when these and other baseline differences were accounted for in the analysis, their mortality in the ensuing 10 years was 61% greater than that of the patients who received an internal mammary artery graft (95% confidence interval, 41%—85% excess). The efficacy of an artery versus a vein graft is supported by:

1. The likelihood that, in the 1970s, the decision to use an artery versus a vein graft had more to do with the person doing the surgery and less to do with the patient's prognosis;
2. The investigators' ability to measure important preoperative predictors of survival, such as left ventricular function;
3. The finding of a large difference in survival after adjusting for the modest differences in preoperative predictors between the 2 groups; and
4. The gradual widening of the survival difference over the course of the 10-year follow-up. Had there been unmeasured differences between recipients of artery and vein grafts that had a strong bearing on survival, they probably would produce a spurious survival disadvantage to vein graft recipients relatively soon after surgery, with the 2 groups' survival curves later becoming parallel.

Comparisons of Nonconcurrent Patient Groups

It is tempting, as a means of increasing between-group comparability, to compare the outcomes of patients given a particular therapy during a recent time period with those of patients treated in a different way in the past. On the surface, an evaluation of this sort would appear to have much to recommend it: In many situations, a greater degree of similarity (in terms of prognostic factors) should be present between 2 groups of patients who are treated at different times than between 2 groups who are seen at the same time but receive different therapies. However, unless the difference in outcome between the groups is substantial, the results of such evaluations are difficult to interpret, given that characteristics relevant to the study outcome may differ in recent and not-so-recent patients. For example, in a 7-year randomized trial of treatment for prostate cancer, it was noted that the annual mortality among patients enrolled in the placebo treatment group in the last several years of the trial was lower than that of patients enrolled in that group in the first several years (Veterans Administration Cooperative Urological Research Group, 1967). Thus, had this not been a randomized trial, and had placebo been replaced by an active therapy in the later time period, an apparent benefit associated with that therapy would have been seen in the absence of any true effect on survival.

Even if an attempt is made to measure and adjust for these patient characteristics (see Question 5.3), it may not be possible to measure comparably some important ones (such as disease severity) in the various time periods, either because of changes in the nature of patient records or because the methods of evaluating patients have changed over time.

Finally, problems in interpretation can be introduced by the fact that ways of caring for patients with a given condition often consist of more than one type of therapy and that these other ways may change over time, as well. So, even if it is felt that there has been a true change in the prognosis of patients with a particular disorder, it may be difficult to ascribe that change to a specific therapeutic agent.

Nonetheless, a large difference in outcome between groups treated in different ways in not-widely-spaced periods of time should not be ignored. For example, of 325 Rh(D)-negative women who received two 100-μg doses of anti-D immunoglobulin in the third trimester of their first pregnancies and another dose at delivery if their infants were Rh(D)-positive, only 2 developed anti-D antibodies in a subsequent Rh(D)-positive pregnancy (Tovey et al., 1983). In contrast, based on the experience of Rh(D)-negative women from the same region who were pregnant in the 2 preceding years and who were treated only at delivery, 18 women in the more recent group would have been expected to develop antibodies. Because little else of consequence had changed with regard to the management of these women, it seems hard to dispute the efficacy of the antenatal prophylaxis.

The administration of some therapeutic agents is followed rapidly by a dramatic favorable change in an individual patient's status. There may be a strong basis for believing that such a change would have been unlikely in the absence of receipt of the agent, perhaps based on the prior experience in that patient or in others. If so, a similar sequence of events seen in only a few such patients constitutes a strong argument that the treatment is truly beneficial. So, for example, the observed improvement in drug-induced allergic symptoms that occurs promptly following parenteral antihistamine therapy—to a degree far greater than would have been expected in the absence of therapy—is a sufficient basis for concluding that this therapy is efficacious.

Nonetheless, unless the change in the patient's status occurs rapidly and reliably in association with a given therapy, it is necessary to be skeptical of the results of within-patient comparisons that are not randomized (Weiss and Heckbert, 1988). Therapies are usually given for a reason—perhaps a chronic symptom has flared up, or a new symptom has just developed—and the course of the patient's condition may soon change for the better in the absence of any therapy at all.

> *Example:* Patients with more than 40 ventricular depolarizations (VPDs) per hour were identified (Pratt et al., 1985). Once it was determined that they were clinically stable, they were simply followed with no active antiarrhythmic treatment. When reevaluated 1–2 years later, their frequency of VPDs was less than 50% that at baseline. Almost certainly, the frequency of VPDs in each patient "regressed" toward its usual, lower, value. Had even an ineffective therapy been administered during the follow-up period, a comparison of the frequency of VPDs before and after its use could have erroneously suggested some antiarrhythmic activity.

> *Example:* In persons who had received immunization against pneumococcal pneumonia, the incidence of pneumonia (of all types) was 69% lower in the year following immunization than in the preceding year (Gable et al., 1990). However, data of this type have little to say regarding the efficacy of pneumococcal vaccine. It is probable that in many of the study subjects, vaccination occurred as an indirect consequence of their having developed pneumonia—for example, in elderly patients the pneumonia could have led to hospitalization, which often can trigger the administration of the vaccine. This process of selection for vaccination would make the occurrence of prior pneumonia in vaccinees anomalously high. Thus, even if the vaccine were completely ineffective, the subsequent rate of pneumonia in vaccinated patients would appear to be relatively low.

Obtaining Comparable Numerators and Denominators between Treatment Groups

Whether a comparison group of patients is concurrent or historical, a strategy to aid in choosing comparable treatment groups is to identify, if possible, a point in the disease process at which the decision to begin (or to continue) the treatment would generally be made. The groups would be defined on the basis of treatment prescribed at that time (and could include 1 group that received no treatment, if such a group were present). The various groups would be compared for the development of disease progression or complications for that period of time over which the treatment plausibly could exert any beneficial effect it might have, and patients would remain as originally grouped even if the therapy were altered later during that period. For example, in a nonrandomized study attempting to evaluate the efficacy of coronary artery bypass surgery, one might identify patients who had undergone their first coronary angiography, some of whom subsequently received surgery (within a predefined time following angiography) and the rest of whom did not. The

2 groups would be compared for, say, mortality from heart disease starting at the time the decision was made to perform surgery and at the equivalent time after angiography for nonsurgical cases. For purposes of analyses, subsequent bypass surgery in the latter group would be disregarded; the patients would remain in the nonsurgical group. Because these late-surgery patients are likely to have a relatively poor prognosis—as indicated by their failure on medical therapy alone—their "transfer" to the group that initially received surgery would spuriously diminish the estimated efficacy of surgical therapy.

Example: In comparing the case fatality between patients who were and were not administered lidocaine, investigators (Horwitz and Feinstein, 1981) were concerned that some patients died so soon after entry to the hospital that lidocaine could not have been ordered, even had a physician wanted to do so. To include these patients in the analysis would be to severely bias the results toward finding a beneficial effect associated with lidocaine. Thus patients who died prior to admission to the hospital's coronary care unit were excluded from the study.

Example: In the analysis of their study of children who had had relapses of acute lymphoblastic leukemia but were presently in remission after chemotherapy, Boulad et al. (1999) wished to compare survival between those who received a bone marrow transplant and those who did not (for lack of a potential marrow donor who was HLA-identical). They recognized that a comparison beginning at the completion of chemotherapy for the relapse would have been biased: Transplants were given an average of 3 months after this time, and then only to children who were believed to still be disease free. So, to increase the validity of the study, the only nontransplant patients entering the analysis were those who were alive and apparently disease free as of 3 months following treatment of their first relapse.

Reminder: Nonrandomized Studies of Efficacy Must Be Interpreted with Caution!

It is easier to stipulate the conditions needed for a nonrandomized study of therapeutic efficacy to provide a valid result—that is, small between-group differences in factors predictive of outcome (confounding factors) either inherently or after manipulation in the study design and/or analysis—than to determine unequivocally whether they are present in a given instance. The only times one can be really "sure" that the between-group differences in confounding factors are small are when the results of randomized trials have corroborated those of the nonrandomized studies, and these are just the times that the nonrandomized studies are the least needed.

Certainly, there are instances in which both randomized and nonrandomized studies of the same therapy have been done and in which similar results have been obtained. For example, tonsillectomy for recurrent throat infection in childhood was associated with roughly the same reduction in the incidence of subsequent infection in a randomized trial and in a parallel study in which parental preference dictated whether surgery was performed (Paradise et al., 1984). Benson and Hartz (2000) and Concato et al. (2000) have provided a number of additional examples of congruence between the results of randomized and nonrandomized studies. However, let's consider an example that is intended to keep us from becoming overconfident in our ability to derive valid comparisons from nonrandomized studies, no matter how hard we strive to achieve comparability of treatment groups:

> *Example:* The results of 6 nonrandomized studies that evaluated the efficacy of anticoagulant drugs in reducing early mortality from acute myocardial infarction were summarized by Sacks et al. (1982). A 17.1% difference in mortality was found (mortality in patients given anticoagulants was 18.0% vs. 35.1% in controls). In 4 of the studies, data were available on some or all of the following prognostic factors: age, sex, location and severity of infarction, history of previous infarction and other diseases. After adjustment for them, the overall mortality difference favoring the anticoagulant-treated group was reduced to 11.0%. Nonetheless, the pooling of data from 10 randomized controlled trials of anticoagulants in acute myocardial infarction revealed a difference of only 3.9% (still favoring the anticoagulant-treated group). Thus the adjustment for prognostic factors that were measured in the nonrandomized studies could in part, but not fully, eliminate the confounding due to underlying differences between patients in the anticoagulant-treated and control groups.

The notion raised in the preceding example—that even after controlling for all measurable, relevant characteristics there could be some hard-to-define characteristic that may vary considerably between the treatment groups and as a result distort the true difference in the measured efficacy of the therapeutic alternatives—has at times received explicit consideration. Mossey and Shapiro (1982) classified a random sample of elderly persons with respect to an index of "objective" health status. The index was based on the presence of certain medical conditions (weighted for severity) and on the degree to which the conditions caused the persons to obtain health care services in the prior year. In addition, the subjects were asked the following question: "For your age would you say, in general, your health is excellent, good, fair, poor?" Mortality rates were monitored in this group ($n = 3,128$) for the next 7 years. Persons who reported their health as "poor" had a mortality rate nearly 3 times that of persons who reported their health as excellent, even after the influence of "objective" health status had been controlled. The message: Although these investigators achieved some success, much of the time we are simply not able to measure (and thus are not able to control for) some important factors that bear on the outcome of the condition for which we are evaluating therapeutic choices. As a consequence, without our knowing it, the treatment groups that are formed in the absence of randomization may be at substantially different risks of the outcome under study.

Integrating Results from Nonrandomized Studies of Therapeutic Efficacy with Other Data

Relatively few randomized controlled trials have been done in humans to help evaluate whether a suspected factor plays an etiologic role in disease occurrence. It is usually far more feasible to conduct a randomized trial of a potential therapeutic agent than a trial of a potential etiologic agent. Thus the question of the adequacy of evidence from nonrandomized studies for inferring cause and effect is addressed often by epidemiologists dealing with the causes of disease. What approaches do they use that are relevant to judging, from data gathering in nonrandomized studies, whether (and to what extent) an agent is effective in treating disease? Apart from the 2 considerations that have been stressed already—the presence of a large difference in outcome between the treatment groups and a small difference in confounding factors—the epidemiologist looks to the plausibility of the cause-and-effect relationship, that is, does it make sense on the basis of other knowledge? Needless to say, the use of this guideline introduces a great deal of subjectivity into the matter, and it is responsible for many disagreements concerning disease etiology, for example the controversies surrounding the possible influence of diet on the incidence of coronary disease and cancer. Still, as hard as it is to apply at times, the question of plausibility cannot be ignored.

Because there is almost always a good reason (pharmacologic, mechanical, nutritional, etc.) for the introduction of most therapeutic measures, the issue of a priori expectation tends to be less useful when applied to therapeutic questions than to etiologic ones. However, the results of nonrandomized studies may suggest that the impact of a particular form of therapy varies across categories of patients or is beneficial for just some illness outcomes and not others. The more the pattern of results obtained in nonrandomized studies of effectiveness corresponds to our expectations based on other information, the stronger the inferences we can make from such studies (Weiss 1981; Weiss, 2002).

> *Example:* Silverstein et al. (1999) monitored the incidence of recurrence among 469 women who had undergone a breast-conserving excision of a ductal carcinoma in situ during the period 1972 through 1998. The 2 institutions at which these women were treated did not have rigid criteria for the use of postoperative radiation therapy in this condition, and the authors indicate that "the patient's preference was important in selecting treatment." For women in whom the minimal margin of tumor-free tissue surrounding the excised lesion was <1 mm, the receipt of radiation therapy was associated with about a 60% re-

duction in the incidence of ipsilateral recurrence, adjusting for other prognostic characteristics such as tumor size and grade. The difference was comparable to that seen in a randomized trial of the same intervention in women with ductal in situ carcinoma (Fisher et al., 2001) but in which an analysis according to margin width was not done. However, among the women in the nonrandomized study whose tumors had a margin width of more than 10 mm, the incidence of recurrence was low (3–4% over 8 years) and nearly identical between women who did and who did not receive postoperative radiation therapy.

Among women whose tumors had been excised with a wide margin, the lack of efficacy of postoperative radiation is supported by:

a. The specificity of this null result: A positive result was seen in women with *narrow* margin widths, just what would have been predicted from the results of randomized trials; and

b. The plausibility of the hypothesis that the benefit from radiation therapy would largely be restricted to women in whom there is a relatively higher likelihood of having some tumor left behind after the initial resection.

Given the very small number of recurrences in the women with margin width > 10 mm in the study of Silverstein et al.—there were only 3 among 133 women in total—it would be premature to conclude that radiation therapy offers no benefit in this circumstance. Nonetheless, it would be reasonable to conclude that because of the underlying low risk of recurrence in these women, the *absolute* benefit associated with radiation therapy could not be large.

Example: In the study mentioned earlier that sought to measure the effect of prophylactic lidocaine on mortality following myocardial infarction (Horwitz and Feinstein, 1981), the investigators categorized each death as being attributable to an arrhythmia or to other causes. The categorization was done without knowledge of whether lidocaine had been administered to the patient. There was about a threefold reduction in mortality from ventricular arrhythmia in the lidocaine-treated group, whereas mortality from other cardiac causes was identical in the 2 groups. The restriction of the mortality reduction to a particular cause of death, especially one that would have been predicted prior to the study to be sensitive to the effect of this medication, makes it less likely that the results could be explained by the tendency for lidocaine to be used selectively in low-risk patients.

Integration of the Results Obtained in Nonrandomized Studies with Those from Randomized Trials

As mentioned in Chapter 4, for reasons of economy and time, randomized trials may be conducted in which the outcome is not the one of greatest interest, but rather a more common "surrogate." If (a) the trials suggest that the treatment in question has a beneficial impact on the surrogate, and (b) there are reasons to believe that the surrogate lies on a pathway linking the treatment and the more relevant outcome, then the results of *non*randomized studies of this more important outcome that suggest a benefit can be relatively convincing.

Example: In case-control studies of postmenopausal women with hip and forearm fractures, the prior use of noncontraceptive estrogens is associated with a decrease in risk, but only if the hormones have been taken for a number of years and have not been discontinued (Weiss et al., 1980; Paganini-Hill et al., 1981; Cauley et al., 1995). Studies of bone density have shown a steadily increasing difference between estrogen-treated and control women over a period of several years (Lindsay et al., 1976), but this difference diminishes or disappears within several years after women have stopped taking the drug (Lindsay et al., 1978). Because the results of the case-control studies "fit" the expectation based on other data, not only as to the overall direction of the effect but also as to the particulars of duration and recency of use, a strong argument could be made for the efficacy of noncontraceptive estrogens in reducing the incidence of fractures, even prior to the conduct of randomized trials of hormone therapy that were large enough to examine fracture risk per se. Ultimately, those trials did observe a reduction in fracture risk associated with administration of hormone therapy (Writing Group for the Women's Health Initiative Investigators, 2002).

Randomized trials often are restricted to subclasses of patients, based on characteristics of the condition being treated (such as severity) or on patient characteristics (such as age). The generalization of the results of randomized trials conducted in one patient subclass to the other(s) can be facilitated by *non*randomized studies of the same question that includes patients not represented in the original trials.

Example: Randomized trials of coronary artery bypass surgery conducted in persons *under* 65 years of age have suggested that, whereas surgery improves survival in some categories of patients, it does not do so among a defined low-risk subset (characterized on the basis of symptoms, signs, and EKG and arteriography results [Braunwald, 1983]). In a nonrandomized follow-up of persons 65 years *and older* with coronary artery disease but who were in the "low-risk" subset, those who underwent bypass surgery had the same mortality rate as persons who received medical therapy alone (Gersh et al., 1985). The concordance of these data with those obtained in the randomized studies of younger patients argues in favor of both (a) not performing bypass surgery in elderly "low-risk" patients with coronary disease and (b) not conducting a randomized trial of bypass surgery in such patients. The results of the nonrandomized study can be used to extend the age range over which the results of the earlier randomized trials can be generalized.

Example: Randomized trials have been conducted to assess the effectiveness of beta blockers given prior to and for a short time after noncardiac surgery (Mangano, 1996). The results of these studies suggest that mortality from cardiac causes is decreased in patients who receive beta blockers, perhaps because the drugs can prevent an exaggerated sympathetic response. Ferguson et al. (2002) asked whether the same benefit might be present in patients undergoing coronary artery bypass graft surgery, using a computerized database that contained information on 629,877 North American patients who underwent this operation during the period 1996–1999. They found that the 30-day postoperative mortality (all causes) in the approximately 55% of persons who received beta blockers prior to surgery was reduced by 6% (95% confidence interval = 3%–9%), after adjusting for characteristics (such as the presence of diabetes and congestive heart failure) that differed between the 2 treatment groups. Although this small difference cannot be interpreted unambiguously as reflecting a true benefit—Ferguson and colleagues themselves recommended that a randomized trial be organized—the likelihood that the difference is genuine is increased by (1) the very large size of the trial and the resulting narrow confidence limits and (2) the observations from the randomized studies of patients undergoing *other* types of surgery that suggest a benefit of beta blocker therapy in reducing mortality.

In a similar way, the results of nonrandomized studies of the effectiveness of a pharmaceutical agent administered at a given dose warrant particular attention if they are consistent with the results of randomized trials of that same agent at a different dose.

Example: It has been documented in randomized trials that, among patients who have sustained a myocardial infarction, the long-term administration of beta blockers is associated with improved survival (Yusuf et al., 1985). However, the daily doses employed in those trials—typically 160 mg of propanolol, 200 mg of metoprolol, or 100 mg of atenolol—commonly produce adverse effects, and, in practice, a number of patients receive lower doses of the agents. Barron et al. (1998) identified 1,050 persons discharged from northern California Kaiser Permanente hospitals during the period 1990–1992, documented the type of beta blocker (if any) and dose prescribed at that time, and monitored this cohort for mortality through the end of 1993. In the group prescribed a beta blocker (*n* = 396), about half were given a dose that was less than 50% that demonstrated in the randomized trials to be effective in reducing mortality. The mortality from cardiovascular disease in these patients was only one-third that of patients who were not prescribed a beta blocker (95% confidence interval = 0.14–0.76), adjusted for demographic characteristics, severity of heart disease, and the degree of comorbidity. The size of the reduced mortality risk associated with prescription of higher doses of beta blockers was not as great (mortality risk relative to nonusers = 0.82, 95% confidence interval = 0.44–1.51), conceivably because of a lower level of compliance with high-dose regimens (though compliance was not assessed in this study). In the absence of a randomized trial that compares the influence of high- and low-dose long-term beta blocker therapy after myocardial infarction, it seems reasonable to conclude that low-dose therapy is indeed efficacious, given the combination of (1) positive results from randomized studies of high-dose therapy and (2) the strong association of low-dose therapy with improved survival in a nonrandomized study that appeared to be well able to address potential confounding.

Actions Based on Results Obtained in Nonrandomized Studies

If a particular therapy has not been evaluated in a randomized trial, but if one or more nonrandomized studies of the efficacy of therapy have been completed, there are 3 general courses of action that a health care provider can take with regard to the therapy:

1. In the nonrandomized studies, the therapy appeared to have no or very little effect, and there were no apparent biases to have nullified a true benefit. *Action:* The therapy should not be used.
2. The results of the nonrandomized studies suggested that the therapy has a great deal of efficacy, far beyond what could reasonably be attributed to possible biases, and this outweighs any known adverse effects. *Action:* The therapy can be put into use (or continue to be used). It is no longer ethical to conduct randomized controlled trials to evaluate the efficacy of this therapy.
3. The therapy appears to have some efficacy, but not beyond what could reasonably be attributed to possible biases. The efficacy, if it were genuine, would outweigh any known adverse effects. *Action:* The therapy could be put into use or could continue to be used (assuming there is no other means of treating the same condition for which there is stronger evidence of efficacy) on an interim basis until the results of randomized controlled trials or more definitive nonrandomized studies are available.

Sometimes the choice among these courses of action is clear-cut. For instance, based on the results obtained in the nonrandomized studies presented earlier, it would be hard to dispute the efficacy of bone marrow transplantation in treating acute lymphoblastic leukemia or, in Rh(D)-negative women, of prepartum anti-D immunoglobulin in preventing the development of anti-D antibodies. Thus most of us would be willing to forgo the requirement of a randomized controlled trial and would not deny either of these therapies to patients for whom they are indicated. In contrast, only the most uncritical would accept as definitive the results of a nonrandomized study of the long-term efficacy of a newly introduced antihypertensive drug, and there would be wide support for a randomized trial to evaluate this form of treatment.

Often the appropriate course of action is less clear. A therapy can appear to be efficacious on the basis of data from nonrandomized studies, but it is uncertain whether the measured efficacy is "far beyond what could reasonably be attributed to possible biases." Gauging the adequacy of data from these studies is very much a subjective process: There are situations in which some persons are certain of a therapy's efficacy, whereas others, reviewing the same evidence, are not. My subjective recommendation is to insist on a very strong demonstration of efficacy in a nonrandomized study before concluding that a randomized controlled trial of the treatment in question is inappropriate. There have been too many examples in which we know we would have been led astray if a controlled trial had not been done. It is true that, if a controlled trial is carried out and it "only" confirms the results of prior nonrandomized studies, the patients enrolled in the trial who were not given the therapy under study would not have benefited as they might have in the absence of the trial. But if the controlled trial is not done and the therapy truly is not efficacious, then a very much larger number of patients will undergo the treatment for no good reason. Indeed, the therapy may actually be detrimental, in which case that very much larger number of patients will be harmed for lack of a controlled trial capable of determining its harmful effect.

> *Example:* During the 1960s in the United States, several drugs were being prescribed to patients who had sustained myocardial infarction in an effort to decrease the likelihood of reinfarction. The evidence supporting the efficacy of these drugs (estrogens, dextrothyroxine, clofibrate, and nicotine acid) was largely or exclusively derived from studies in which randomization had not been done. A group of investigators judged this evidence to be less than definitive, and they mounted a large randomized controlled trial—the Coronary Drug Project—to evaluate more thoroughly whether the use of one of these drugs could truly reduce the rate of reinfarction.
>
> The results of this study were disappointing, to put it mildly. Relative to the subjects given a placebo, those given clofibrate experienced no reduction in mortality from coronary disease, and those given estrogens or dextrothyroxine actually experienced an increase (Coronary Drug Project Research Group, 1970, 1972, 1973, 1975). In the United States, the use of these drugs among patients in the postinfarction period declined precipitously following the publication of these results (Friedman et al., 1983).

Which Type of Nonrandomized Design to Choose?

Given that you are going to try to measure the efficacy of a therapy without the benefit of a randomized trial, which nonrandomized approach—cohort or case control—is preferable? The intuitive choice, one that works well in many situations, is the cohort approach: Patients treated in different ways are monitored and compared with respect to the rate of disease progression or complications. However, if (a) a relatively small fraction (less than 10% or so) of patients develops the progression/complications during the planned period of follow-up, (b) it is necessary to obtain a considerable amount of information on each study subject (e.g., related to the assessment of disease severity), and (c) the use of the therapy itself is not too uncommon among patients with the condition, it may prove far more economical to do a case-control study. This would involve identifying persons in whom the progression/complications occurred and a sample of patients in whom these did not occur. The treatment given to members of each of the 2 groups would be ascertained, along with characteristics known to influence the rate of progression/complications. The greater the degree to which "cases" (i.e., patients who develop progression/complications) have received a therapeutic measure less often than controls, the greater the efficacy of that measure (see Chapter 6 for more on the analysis of and inferences from case-control studies).

Example: A study of the comparative efficacy of various antihypertensive agents used a case-control design (Psaty et al., 1995). Among hypertensive members of a prepaid health care plan who sustained a first myocardial infarction ("cases"), medical and pharmacy records were reviewed to determine which treatment(s) the patient had been undergoing and what risk factors for myocardial infarction had been present. Records also were reviewed for a sample of hypertensive patients who had not sustained a myocardial infarction, chosen in such a way as to be comparable to the cases with respect to age and gender. Type and dose of the antihypertensive agent(s) used were compared between the 2 groups, both overall and after excluding persons with evidence of prior heart disease. The investigators chose a case-control approach because a myocardial infarction occurred in but a small minority of patients during the period of the study and because of the time required to extract data from the chart of each one.

Questions

5.1. In the mid-1970s, concern over the safety of pertussis vaccine led a number of British physicians not to administer it in its typical combination with diphtheria and tetanus vaccines (DPT vaccine) but instead to use diphtheria/tetanus (DT) vaccine. From January 1978 through June 1980, pertussis cases were identified in 21 English "health areas," and the incidence of pertussis was tabulated as a function of type of vaccine received (Pollock et al., 1982). The results were as follows: 2,261 cases of pertussis in 250,163 children vaccinated with DPT, and 9,515 cases of pertussis in 187,595 children vaccinated with DT.

a. What was the incidence of pertussis during this 2.5-year period in the group that received DPT vaccine? In the group that received DT vaccine?

b. Does it seem likely that the disparity between these rates could be attributed to differences in the characteristics of the children who received the 2 vaccines?

5.2. The following abstract (condensed and somewhat modified) appeared in a prominent journal in the mid-1990s:

> *Objective:* To investigate the relation between suboptimal intrapartum obstetric care and intrapartum or neonatal death.
> *Design:* Case-control study.
> *Subjects:* Sixty babies who died intrapartum or neonatally. All were the products of singleton pregnancies and had no congenital anomaly. Two controls, matched for place and time of birth, were selected for each index case.
> *Main outcome measures:* Adverse antenatal factors and suboptimal intrapartum care (by using predefined criteria) identified through the use of medical records without knowledge of case-control status.
> *Results:* Failure of providers of obstetric care to respond to signs of severe fetal distress was more common in the children who died (50%) than among controls (6.9%). This association persisted even after adjustment for the presence of antenatal characteristics predisposing to complications of labor and delivery (e.g., pre-eclampsia, oligo- or polyhydramnios, previous poor obstetric history).
> *Conclusion:* There is an association between the quality of intrapartum care and death.

You are concerned that the association noted in the conclusion may not represent a causal one. Why? How could this case-control study have been designed so as to have diminished your concern?

5.3. You are a gynecologist at a large medical center and you would like to evaluate your institution's past success in treating ovarian cancer. You have data for patients from 2 periods, 1965–1975 and 1985–1995, and you wish to determine whether patient survival improved over the interval. Therapy for ovarian cancer had changed considerably, with radiation therapy and promising chemotherapeutic agents being used to a larger extent from 1985 to 1995. Procedures to evaluate the patients were similar between the 2 periods, except that thorough surgical assessment was employed considerably more often to detect the spread of ovarian cancer during 1985 through 1995.

Because you are aware of the relationship between histologic type and survival, you obtain survival data specific for serous cystadenocarcinomas alone. Following are the (hypothetical) data obtained:

Stage (when first treated at the medical center)	1965–1975			1985–1995		
	No. of subjects	No. of 5-year survivors	% 5-year survival	No. of subjects	No. of 5-year survivors	% 5-year survival
I (spread limited to ovaries)	30	18	60	20	14	70
II (spread limited to pelvic structures)	50	20	40	40	20	50
III, IV (spread beyond pelvic structures)	20	0	0	40	4	10

In the period 1965–1975, 38 of the 100 women survived for at least 5 years (18 women with Stage I disease and 20 women with Stage II disease). In the 100 women treated during the period 1985–1995, there were also 38 five-year survivors (14 + 20 + 4 among women with Stage I, II, and III disease, respectively). However, by adjusting for stage—that is, by analytically "forcing" the stage distribution to be identical in each time period—a different result emerges. If the 1965–1975 patients had had the stage distribution of the 1985–1995 patients, the expected number of survivors would be as follows:

Stage I	60% × 20	= 12
Stage II	40% × 40	= 16
Stage III	0% × 40	= 0
Total		28

Thus an analysis that adjusts for stage of disease suggests that for every 100 women with ovarian cancer treated during 1985–1995, there were 10 additional survivors (38−28) compared with the earlier era.

a. Why does the size of the difference in 5-year survival between the 2 time periods depend on whether or not adjustment was performed?

b. What assumptions are needed in order to decide which of the 2 sets of results, adjusted or unadjusted, offers a more valid portrait of the true difference in survival from serous cystadenocarcinoma of the ovary between the 2 time periods?

5.4. The presence of a cryptorchid (undescended) testis increases by a factor of 5–10 a man's risk of testicular cancer. Because surgical correction of this abnormality prior to puberty is associated with a reduced occurrence of degenerative changes in the cryptorchid testis, it is suspected that such correction might prevent some cases of cancer.

Although testicular cancer is the most commonly occurring malignancy in young adult men, its incidence in 20- to 40-year-old men is only about 1 per 10,000 per year and is lower at older ages.

a. A randomized controlled trial to determine the efficacy of correction of cryptorchidism at various ages (e.g., <5 years, >5 years) in reducing the risk of testicular cancer has never been done, and probably never will be. Why is this?

b. What type of nonrandomized study would be the most practical in addressing this question? Specifically, what groups should be compared?

c. To what extent would the results of such a nonrandomized study be credible, in view of the confounding that often plagues nonrandomized studies of therapeutic efficacy?

5.5. Using data from U.S. end-stage renal disease networks, an effort was made to measure the relative impact of renal transplant and dialysis on survival (Krakauer et al., 1983). In patients receiving dialysis, mortality rates were monitored from the initiation of dialysis until the end of the follow-up period, or until a transplant had been received. Mortality among transplant recipients was monitored from the time of transplant until the end of the follow-up period, unless the transplant was rejected, in which case follow-up ceased (for purposes of this analysis) 90 days after the rejection.

This comparison had the potential to distort any true difference between the respective effects of transplant and dialysis on survival of patients with end-stage renal disease. Why? How should the mortality comparison have been made to remove this possible distortion?

5.6. In 1994, a randomized controlled trial observed that zidovudine (AZT) given antepartum, intrapartum, and to the newborn was associated with a reduction in the perinatal transmission of HIV infection from 25.5% to 8.3%. In New York State during the period 1995–1997, AZT was recommended for HIV-positive women who were pregnant. However, "abbreviated regimens . . . were used as a result of the lack of or limited prenatal care or maternal choice." The following table summarizes the results of a study that examined the occurrence of HIV infection in infants of HIV-infected mothers in relation to the time of initiation of AZT prophylaxis (Wade et al., 1998).

Time of initiation of AZT prophylaxis	No. of infants (%)	Positive test for HIV	Relative risk (95% confidence interval)
Prenatal	423	26	0.23 (0.16–0.34)
Intra-partum	50	5	0.38 (0.18–0.81)
Within 48 hr after birth	86	8	0.35 (0.19–0.65)
>3 Days after birth (up to 42 days)	38	7	0.69 (0.35–1.36)
No AZT prophylaxis	237	63	1.0 (referent category)

The relative risks shown in the table were influenced to only a small degree by adjustment for race, sex, and birth weight. Based on these observations, the authors concluded: "Women who do not receive zidovudine during pregnancy [should be] identified so that they can receive antiretroviral prophylaxis during delivery and their infants can begin receiving zidovudine soon after birth."

However, an editorial that accompanied the article by Wade and colleagues warned: "There must inevitably be uncertainty about the results of a retrospective observational study such as this one. For example, bias could have crept into the study because of rapidly changing obstetrical practices in the care of HIV-infected women during the two years of the survey."

a. What are the 2 circumstances that must be true for bias from this source to have occurred?

b. Do you think both of these are likely to have been present to any appreciable degree?

c. If they were permitted to respond to the editorial, what could the authors of the study do to address the concern?

5.7. The following question pertains to the abstract (slightly abridged) of an article titled "Aspirin and Mortality from Coronary Bypass Surgery" (Magano et al., 2002):

> *Background:* Because platelet activation constitutes a pivotal mechanism for injury in patients with atherosclerosis, we assessed whether early treatment with aspirin could improve survival after coronary bypass surgery.
> *Methods:* At 70 centers in 17 countries, we prospectively studied 5,065 patients undergoing coronary bypass surgery, of whom 5,022 survived the first 48 hours after surgery. The primary focus was to discern the relation between early aspirin use and fatal and nonfatal outcomes.
> *Results:* Among patients who received aspirin (up to 650 mg) within 48 hours after revascularization, subsequent mortality was 1.3% (40 of 2,999 patients), as compared with 4.0% among those who did not receive aspirin during this period (81 of 2,023, $P < 0.001$). Aspirin therapy was associated with a 48% reduction in the incidence of myocardial infarction (2.8% vs. 5.4%, $P < 0.001$), a 50% reduction in the incidence of stroke (1.3% vs. 2.6%, $P = 0.01$), a 74% reduction in the incidence of renal failure (0.9% vs. 3.4%, $P < 0.001$), and a 62% reduction in the incidence of bowel infarction (0.3% vs. 0.8%, $P = 0.01$).
> *Conclusions:* Early use of aspirin after coronary bypass surgery is safe and is associated with a reduced risk of death and ischemic complications involving the heart, brain, kidneys and gastrointestinal tract.

The reduced risk of death and the other adverse outcomes listed persisted after adjustment for other measured characteristics that plausibly were associated with these outcomes.

An accompanying editorial stated that this "report might actually underestimate the benefit of early aspirin use (since) the deaths that occurred in the first 48 hours after coronary bypass surgery were not included in the analysis." Those deaths occurred in 41 of 2,064 patients who did not receive aspirin during the first 48 hours and in only 2 of 3,001 patients who did.

The risk of death among patients who received aspirin was only 3% (2/3001) / (41/2064) that of patients who did not, a relative risk far lower than that seen beginning 48 hours after surgery. Yet in their analysis the authors of the study ignored, properly, these deaths that occurred during the first 48 hours. What do you believe to have been their rationale?

Answers

5.1.a. The cumulative incidence of pertussis in the DPT-vaccinated group was 2,261/250,163 = 903.8 per 100,000; and, in the DT-vaccinated group, 9,515/187,595 = 5,072.1 per 100,000.

b. There was a greater than fivefold difference in the incidence of pertussis between the 2 groups of children. To judge whether the difference might have been due to something other than the effect of the vaccine, it is necessary to consider the other factors that bear on the incidence of pertussis and to what extent they may differ between the DPT- and DT-vaccinated groups. "Host" factors appear to be relatively unimportant in pertussis—most nonimmunized persons exposed to the pathogen develop the disease. In any event, it is hard to imagine how the reasons for choosing DT over DPT vaccine, reasons relating to physician and/or parental concern over possible adverse affects, could relate in an important way to a child's underlying risk of pertussis. Thus it would seem safe to conclude from this nonrandomized study that most, if not all, of the difference in pertussis incidence between DPT- and DT-vaccinated groups was due to the use of the pertussis vaccine.

5.2. In order for there to be a failure to respond to severe fetal distress, there must first *be* fetal distress! Such distress would have been present far more often in the infants who died than in other infants born at the same place and time, even after adjustment for factors that predispose to complications of labor and delivery. Therefore, even if failure to respond to fetal distress truly had no bearing on the likelihood of survival, it would have been encountered more frequently in the case group than in the control group.

A case-control study with a greater likelihood of obtaining a valid result would have restricted both cases and controls to those infants who had evidence of fetal distress and then would have measured and adjusted for the severity of such distress when comparing the intrapartum care administered to the 2 groups.

5.3.a. The difference in 5-year survival between the 2 time periods is 0 before adjustment and 10 per 100 after adjustment for stage. This results from the fact that the stage distribution among the cases in the 2 time periods was quite different—there being a higher proportion of more advanced stages during the 1985–1995 period—and from the strong relationship between stage and 5-year survival. When the stage distribution is forced (via adjustment) to be the same in the 2 time periods, the difference of 10 per 100 women in stage-specific 5-year survival that favors the recent time period is reflected in the overall survival.

b. If the difference in stage distribution between the 2 time periods is real, then it is essential to adjust for stage because the higher proportion of more serious cases in the 1985–1995 period (perhaps due to changes in patterns of referral to the medical center) in an unadjusted comparison would result in bias against finding any improvement in 5-year survival over time.

But is it possible that there has been no real change in the stage distribution, that the apparent difference is due to the fact that stage was not evaluated the same way in 1985–1995 as it was 20 years earlier? Yes: Had thorough surgical assessment been conducted during the 1965–1975 period as often as it had been during the period 1985–1995, some women's tumors that were categorized as Stage I at the time would have been correctly categorized as Stages II–IV. The remaining women with "true" Stage I tumors would have had a better survival than would women in the original group that contained the miscategorized cases, because they, on the average, had less extensive disease.

And what would happen to the mean survival of women with Stage II–IV tumors once the "former" Stage I cases, now correctly classified, were included? It is likely that it would be greater as well because of the presence of women with less obvious tumor extension; overall, the group would have a better chance of survival than the original group of Stage II–IV cases.

Therefore, it is possible that, even with no change in the effectiveness of therapy over the 2 decades, a change in the way in which stage was determined could have produced an increase in the stage-specific survival (and thus the stage-adjusted survival). Without knowing to what extent the change in stage distribution was due to a true difference in the distribution of disease severity rather than to an altered way of identifying "stage" itself, no conclusion can be reached concerning improvement in the efficacy of therapy.

5.4.a. It is not feasible to conduct a randomized trial of a treatment that would require enrollment of the necessary tens of thousands of individuals with a relatively uncommon condition (such as cryptorchid testis), particularly if the follow-up period required exceeds 15 years (i.e., from before age 5 through beyond age 20).

b. Given the relative rarity of testicular cancer, a case-control approach generally will be the most feasible. Among men with a history of cryptorchid testis, those with and without testicular cancer would be compared with regard to their history of orchiopexy. The data obtained might be displayed as follows:

Men with a history of cryptorchid testis

Orchiopexy	Cases of testicular cancer	Controls (no testicular cancer)
No	a	d
Yes, >5 years old	b	e
Yes, <5 years old	c	f

The efficacy of orchiopexy before 5 years of age would be supported to the extent that the ratio of $f : d$ exceeded $c : a$. Several studies have now examined the possible efficacy of orchiopexy in this way (Pottern et al., 1985; Strader et al., 1988).

c. The results of these studies would be credible if there were reasons to believe that those factors influencing the occurrence of orchiopexy at an early age did not have some bearing on the incidence of testicular cancer. Among cryptorchid males, the only known such factor is the number of undescended testes, the risk being particularly high in men with a history of bilateral cryptorchidism. Therefore, if the analysis were done separately in men with a history of unilateral and bilateral nondescent, the results would not have any obvious source of bias due to confounding.

5.5. Once a transplant has taken place, it is necessary to consider all deaths that occur during the whole of the follow-up period, whether or not the transplant has been rejected. It is possible, for example, that the likelihood of survival among transplant recipients is less among those who have rejected the transplant than among those who have not and that this reduced survival extends beyond the first 90 days after rejection. If so, even if dialysis and transplant truly had the same influence on mortality, the group undergoing dialysis would appear to have a poorer prognosis in the analysis that was done—no subgroup of dialysis patients who had a high mortality risk comparable to that of the transplant rejectees would have been excluded.

5.6.a(i). The proportion of HIV-infected pregnant women and their infants who received abbreviated regimens, relative to the proportion who received no AZT, must have varied over time during the 2 years; *and*

a(ii). The obstetrical practices that changed during the 2 years must have had an impact on the likelihood of perinatal HIV transmission.

b. If the receipt of an abbreviated AZT regimen versus no AZT therapy were truly dictated primarily by the timing of the onset of prenatal care or maternal choice, it seems unlikely that the proportion of women receiving an abbreviated regimen would have varied appreciably during the period of the study. Thus, even if effective obstetrical practices against perinatal transmission had been introduced during the 2 years, there would have been little or no confounding from this source.

c. The authors could have adjusted for date of delivery.

5.7. Among coronary artery bypass patients, it may be that those with an inherently better prognosis tend to be prescribed aspirin during the first 48 hours following surgery. Indeed, some intraoperative or early postoperative deaths take place before aspirin can be administered. In other words, death can be a cause of nonuse of aspirin.

References

Barron HV, Viskin S, Lundstrom RJ, et al. B-Blocker dosages and mortality after myocardial infarction. *Arch Intern Med* 1998;158:449–453.

Boulad F, Steinherz P, Reyes B, et al. Allogeneic bone marrow transplantation versus chemotherapy for the treatment of childhood acute lymphoblastic leukemia in second remission: A single-institution study. *J Clin Oncol* 1999;17:197–207.

Benson K, Hartz AJ. A comparison of observational studies and randomized, controlled trials. *N Engl J Med* 2000;342:1878–1886.

Braunwald E. Effect of coronary-artery bypass grafting on survival. *N Engl J Med* 1983;309:1181–1184.

Broome CV, Facklamm RR, Fraser DW. Pneumococcal disease after pneumococcal vaccination. *N Engl J Med* 1980;303:549–552.

Cauley JA, Seeley DG, Ensrud K, et al. Estrogen replacement therapy and fractures in older women. *Ann Intern Med* 1995;122:9–16.

Concato J, Shah N, Horwitz RI. Randomized, controlled trials, observational studies, and the hierarchy of research designs. *N Engl J Med* 2000;342:1887–1892.

Coronary Drug Project Research Group. The Coronary Drug Project: Findings leading to further modification of its protocol. *JAMA* 1970;214:1303–1313.

Coronary Drug Project Research Group. The Coronary Drug Project: Findings leading to further modification of its protocol with respect to dexthrothyroxine. *JAMA* 1972;220:966–1008.

Coronary Drug Project Research Group. The Coronary Drug Project: Findings leading to discontinuation of the 2.5 mg/day estrogen group. *JAMA* 1973;226:652–657.

Coronary Drug Project Research Group. Clofibrate and niacin in coronary heart disease. *JAMA* 1975;231:360–381.

Ferguson TB, Coombs LP, Peterson E. Preoperative B-Blocker use and mortality and morbidity following CABG surgery in North America. *JAMA* 2002;287:2221–2227.

Fisher B, Land S, Mamounas E, et al. Prevention of invasive breast cancer in women with ductal carcinoma in situ: An update of the National Surgical Adjuvant Breast and Bowel Project experience. *Sem Oncol* 2001;28:400–418.

Friedman L, Wenger NK, Knatterrud GL. Impact of the coronary drug project findings on clinical practice. *Controlled Clin Trials* 1983;4:515–522.

Gable CB, Holzer SS, Engelhart L, et al. Pneumococcal vaccine: Efficacy and associated cost savings. *JAMA* 1990;264:2910–2915.

Gersh BJ, Kronmal RA, Schaff HV, et al. Comparison of coronary artery bypass surgery and medical therapy in patients 65 years of age or older. *N Engl J Med* 1985;313:217–224.

Horwitz RI, Feinstein AR. Improved observational method for studying therapeutic efficacy: Suggestive evidence that lidocaine prophylaxis prevents death in acute myocardial infarction. *JAMA* 1981;246:2455–2459.

Johnson FL, Thomas ED, Clark BS, et al. A comparison of marrow transplantation with chemotherapy for children with acute lymphoblastic leukemia in second or subsequent remission. *N Engl J Med* 1981;305–846—851.

Kauff ND, Satagopan JM, Robson ME, et al. Risk-reducing salpingo-oophorectomy in women with a *BRCA*1 or *BRCA*2 mutation. *N Engl J Med* 2002;346:1609–1615.

Krakauer H, Grauman JS, McMullan MR, et al. The recent U. S. experience in the treatment of end-stage renal disease by dialysis and transplantation. *N Engl J Med* 1983;308:1558–1563.

Lindsay R, Aitken JM, Anderson JB, et al. Long-term prevention of postmenopausal osteoporosis by estrogen: Evidence for an increased bone mass after delayed onset of estrogen treatment. *Lancet* 1976;1:1038–1040.

Lindsay R, MacLean A, Kraszewski A, et al. Bone response to termination of oestrogen treatment. *Lancet* 1978;1:1325–1327.

Loop FD, Lytle BW, Cosgrove DM, et al. Influence of the internal-mammary-artery graft on 10-year survival and other cardiac events. *N Engl J Med* 1986;314:1–6.

Mangano DT, for the Multicenter Study of Perioperative Ischemia Research Group. Aspirin and mortality from coronary bypass surgery. *N Engl J Med* 2002;347:1309–1317.

Mangano DT, Layug EL, Wallace A, et al. Effect of atenolol on mortality and cardiovascular morbidity after noncardiac surgery. *N Engl J Med* 1996;335:1713–1720.

Monson RR, MacMahon B, Austin JH. Postoperative irradiation in carcinoma of the endometrium. *Cancer* 1973;31:630–632.

Mossey JM, Shapiro E. Self-rated health; A predictor of mortality among the elderly. *Am J Public Health* 1982;72:800–808.

Naumann RW. The role of radiation therapy in early endometrial cancer. *Curr Opin Obstet Gynecol* 2002;14:75–79.

Paganini-Hill A, Ross RK, Gerkins VR, et al. Menopausal estrogen therapy and hip fractures. *Ann Intern Med* 1981;95:28–31.

Paradise JL, Bluestone CD, Bachman RZ, et al. Efficacy of tonsillectomy for recurrent throat infection in severely affected children. *N Engl J Med* 1984;301:674–683.

Pocock SJ, Elbourne DR. Randomized trials or observational tribulations? *N Engl J Med* 2000;342:1907–1909.

Pollock TM, Miller F, Lobb J, et al. Efficacy of pertussis vaccination in England. *Br Med J* 1982;285:357–359.

Pottern LM, Brown LM, Hoover RN, et al. Testicular cancer risk among young men: Role of cryptorchidism and inguinal hernia. *J Natl Cancer Institute* 1985;74:377–381.

Pratt CM, Delclos G, Wierman AM, et al. The changing base line of complex ventricular arrhythmias. *N Engl J Med* 1985;313:1444–1449.

Psaty BM, Heckbert SR, Koepsell TD, et al. The risk of myocardial infarction associated with antihypertensive drug therapies. *JAMA* 1995;274:620–625.

Psaty BM, Koepsell TD, Siscovick D, et al. An approach to several problems in using large databases for population-based case-control studies of the therapeutic efficacy and safety of anti-hypertensive medicines. *Stat Med* 1991;10:653–662.

Rebbeck TR, Lynch HT, Neuhausen SL, et al. Prophylactic oophorectomy in carriers of *BRCA1* or *BRCA2* mutations. *N Engl J Med* 2002;346:1616–1622.

Sacks H, Chalmers TC, Smith H. Randomized versus historical controls for clinical trials. *Am J Med* 1982;72:233–239.

Schimpf K, Brackmann HH, Kreuz W, et al. Absence of anti-human immunodeficiency virus types 1 and 2 seroconversion after the treatment of hemophilia A or V on Willebrand's disease with pasteurized factor VIII concentrate. *N Engl J Med* 1989;321:1148–1152.

Silverstein MJ, Lagios MD, Groshen S, et al. The influence of margin width on local control of ductal carcinoma in situ of the breast. *N Engl J Med* 1999;340:1455–1461.

Strader CH, Weiss NS, Daling JR, et al. Cryptorchism, orchiopexy, and the risk of testicular cancer. *Am J Epidemiol* 1988;127:1013–1018.

Tovey LAD, Townley A, Stevenson BJ, et al. The Yorkshire antenatal anti-D immunoglobulin trial in primigravadae. *Lancet* 1983;2:244–246.

Veterans Administration Cooperative Urological Research Group. Treatment and survival of patients with cancer of the prostate. *Surg Gynecol Obstet* 1967;124:1011–1017.

Vollmer WM, Wahl PW, Blagg CR. Survival with dialysis and transplantation in patients with end-stage renal disease. *N Engl J Med* 1983;308:1553–1558.

Wade NA, Birkhead GS, Warren BL, et al. Abbreviated regimens of Zidovudine prophylaxis and perinatal transmission of the human immunodeficiency virus. *N Engl J Med* 1998;339:1409–1414.

Weiss NS. Inferring causal relationships: Elaboration of the criterion of "dose-response." *Am J Epidemiol* 1981;113:487–490.

Weiss NS. Can the "specificity" of an association be rehabilitated as a basis for supporting a causal hypothesis? *Epidemiology* 2002;13:6–8

Weiss NS, Heckbert SR. Patients as their own controls in studies of therapeutic efficacy. *J Gen Intern Med* 1988;3:381–383.

Weiss NS, Ure CL, Ballard JH, et al. Decreased risk of fractures of the hip and lower forearm with postmenopausal use of estrogen. *N Engl J Med* 1980;303:1195–1198.

Writing Group for the Women's Health Initiative Investigators. Risks and benefits of estrogen plus progestin in healthy postmenopausal women: Principal results from the Women's Health Initiative randomized controlled trial. *JAMA* 2002;288:321–333.

Yusuf S, Peto R, Lewis J, et al. Beta blockade during and after myocardial infarction: An overview of the randomized trials. *Prog Cardiovasc Dis* 1985;27:335–71.

6

Therapeutic Safety

Role of Randomized Controlled Trials

We have seen the heavy reliance that is placed on results of randomized trials in evaluating the efficacy of a given therapy. Unfortunately, randomized trials cannot contribute as much to our understanding of the adverse effects associated with these same therapies. Randomized controlled trials usually are based on samples of several dozen to several thousand subjects. Some adverse effects that bear heavily on a therapy's risk/benefit ratio are relatively uncommon and so may not occur in any one study. Even if certain adverse experiences do occur among the study subjects and differ in frequency between the treated and untreated groups, their frequency may be too low to exclude chance as an explanation.

Figure 6.1 relates the difference in the cumulative frequency of a particular adverse event between treatment and control groups (the groups are assumed to be of equal size) to the number of subjects needed to reliably identify its association with treatment. The figure indicates that a study is unlikely to detect with any degree of precision small, true, absolute differences in the frequencies of an adverse event between 2 groups unless a very large number of subjects are enrolled. For example, it would be necessary to study nearly 1,000 treated patients to document an adverse event that manifests itself in 1% of them, even if the occurrence of this event in the untreated patients were only one tenth as great. The more common the event in the untreated patients (e.g., the upper line in Figure 6.1), the larger must be the study to detect a difference of a given absolute magnitude. Thus it is no surprise that the

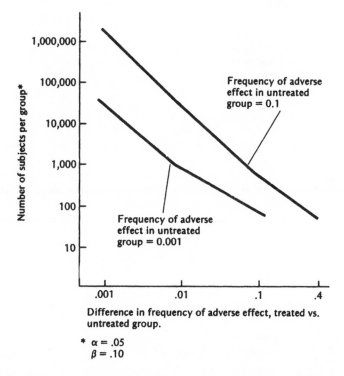

Figure 6.1 Influences of the size of the difference to be detected and the frequency of the adverse effect in the untreated group on the number of subjects needed in a randomized trial.

excess risk of vaginal adenocarcinoma caused by in utero diethylstilbestrol (DES) exposure, estimated from a cohort study to be not more than 1 per 1,000 (Lanier et al., 1973), would not be documented in the follow-up of the daughters of the several hundred women who participated in the clinical trials of this drug (Bibbo et al., 1977; Beral and Colwell, 1981). Indeed, not a single case appeared in the latter studies.

Here are some examples to help us get a feeling for the conditions that are needed for randomized trials to succeed in identifying uncommon adverse effects.

Example: Investigators at the National Cancer Institute were concerned with the possible adverse effects of alkylating agents administered in the treatment of ovarian cancer (Greene et al., 1982). From data collected in 5 separate randomized trials, in which a total of 1,399 subjects were enrolled, they monitored the subsequent incidence of acute leukemia. In the 998 women who received alkylating agents, 12 cases of leukemia occurred. Only 0.11 cases would have been expected on the basis of leukemia incidence rates among women in general, and no cases of leukemia were found in the 401 women to whom alkylating agents were not given. This investigation was successful in document-ing the high risk of leukemia because the excess risk associated with the administration of alkylating agents was indeed great, elevated by more than 100 times, and because the investigators were able to aggregate a large enough body of data so that they could virtually rule out the role of chance in producing the excess.

Example: To evaluate the role of systemic corticosteroid therapy in producing peptic ulcers, results were pooled from 71 randomized con-trolled trials in which the occurrence of side effects was monitored (Messer et al., 1983). Fifty-five (1.8%) of the 3,064 steroid-treated pa-tients developed ulcers, significantly more than the 0.8% of 2,897 con-trols ($p < 0.05$). Had the data set been smaller, this increase in risk for an infrequent adverse effect would have been "missed" (i.e., the same difference in incidence between the 2 groups could have been more plausibly attributed to chance).

The duration of use of a therapy in a randomized trial is often limited. For example, a comparison of lovastatin and cholestyramine resin treatment of severe hypercholesterolemia involved 12 participating centers that ran-domized 264 patients to receive one of these agents (Lovastatin Study Group III, 1988). The duration of treatment was 12 weeks, and every 2 weeks study participants were queried regarding symptoms they were experiencing. A dif-ference in the occurrence of symptoms related to the gastrointestinal tract—58% of patients receiving cholestyramine versus only about 14% of patients receiving lovastatin—was clearly evident in the study. However, because the trial concluded after 12 weeks, any untoward events that arose after longer term treatment would not have been evident. Certainly, some adverse effects of other therapies are of this type. For example, retinopathy from the use of chloroquine generally develops only after 3 years of use (Bernstein, 1967). Only a small minority of randomized trials continue for more than 3 years.

Some important adverse effects may not be manifest until long after drug use has ceased. Thus the excess incidence of vaginal adenocarcinoma in girls who were exposed in utero to DES, appearing some 15 years after exposure, could not be detected in trials that evaluated the effects of DES on the imme-diate outcome of pregnancy.

Finally, there are some adverse effects of a therapeutic agent whose occur-rence may be influenced as much by the manner in which it is delivered as by the agent itself. Thus it is possible that the experience generated in random-ized trials regarding the incidence of a potential adverse effect may not mirror that incidence when the therapy is in general use. For example, it has been suggested that the occurrence of major hemorrhage observed in patients ran-domized to receive the anticoagulant warfarin—1.3 per 100 per year, about 0.3 per 100 more than in placebo recipients—is likely to "underestimate the true risk of hemorrhage in clinical practice [since] the mechanisms used by these trials to monitor anticoagulation may be more reliable than those used in routine practice" (Stern et al., 2000).

Role of Nonrandomized Studies

In view of the limitations of randomized trials in the area of therapeutic safety, it is fortunate that nonrandomized studies can generally be trusted to provide more valid answers in this area than they can for drug efficacy. Why is this so? The reason is that the presence of a given symptom or condition that leads to the use of a particular treatment is often unrelated to the likelihood of the patient's developing the adverse effect in question. For example, the decision to use chloroquine prophylaxis is based on considerations other than the patient's proclivity to develop retinopathy, so a comparison of the frequency of retinopathy in users and nonusers probably will be a valid one. This contrasts with the decidedly limited validity of a nonrandomized comparison of chloroquine users' and nonusers' rates of developing malaria; in these cases, it is likely that users of the drug would be those persons at highest risk of the disease, for instance, persons traveling to or residing in areas of highest disease transmission.

Case Reports and Case Series

Sometimes a health care provider perceives that an unusual manifestation has occurred in a patient given a certain type of treatment. He or she might take note of it and might be prompted to look for a similar manifestation in subsequent similarly treated patients and may report the possibility of an etiologic connection to colleagues or to an appropriate agency (such as the MedWatch program of the U.S. Food and Drug Administration; http://www.fda.gov/medwatch/index.html). This is the manner by which many untoward effects of therapy first come under suspicion, whether they may be infection following certain types of surgical procedures or anaphylaxis following administration of a drug (Wysowski and Swartz, 2005). If there are substantial numbers of reported instances of an otherwise quite uncommon condition—such as the hundreds of reports of hepatic injury in users of the diuretic ticrynofen that led to withdrawal of this drug from the market within 1 year of its introduction (Zimmerman et al., 1984)—formal pharmacoepidemiologic study of the question may not be necessary to form a judgment of a cause-effect relation. In other circumstances, a comparison of adverse events reported for different drugs with a similar indication and similar time of entry into the market, combined with sales data on the drugs, can be informative. For example, the nearly hundredfold higher frequency of reports of rhabdomyolysis in users of cerivastatin than in users of atorvastatin, taking into account the estimated number of users of each drug, provided compelling evidence of a particular hazard associated with use of cerivastatin (Staffa et al., 2002).

Nonetheless, it is apparent that the specificity and sensitivity of this sort of reporting "system" is poor. First, such reports identify far more potential associations than would be verified if more detailed studies could be done to corroborate the relationships. Second, some bona fide adverse effects will not be reported as such, particularly if the incidence of the adverse effect is low, if the effect does not promptly follow administration of therapy, or if the effect is more commonly caused by factors other than the therapy in question. For example, more than 40 years elapsed between the time estrogens were first used in the treatment of menopausal symptoms and the time that studies using controls were done to document the association of such use with the increased incidence of endometrial cancer. Recognition was delayed because, in part, (a) most estrogen users did not develop endometrial cancer, (b) there was an interval of several years between first use and the appearance of excess risk of the disease, and (c) the occurrence of endometrial cancer in a postmenopausal woman is not uncommon even in the absence of exogenous estrogens.

Clearly, what is needed to evaluate therapeutic safety is the determination of the rate of the particular manifestation suspected to be an unintended effect, both in persons who have and have not received the therapy.[1] The nonrandomized studies that make these comparisons are (a) cohort (follow-up) studies, which estimate the rates directly, and (b) case-control studies, which allow the estimation of relative rates.

Cohort (Follow-Up) Studies

Cohort studies first characterize persons as to whether or not they have received a particular therapy and then monitor them for the occurrence of one or more symptoms, signs, or illnesses that could represent an adverse effect. The monitoring can be prospective in persons currently being treated or retrospective, so that persons treated in the past can be monitored until the time of the study.

An example of the *prospective* approach is the follow-up, for mortality, of patients to whom cimetidine was prescribed (Colin-Jones et al., 1983). These patients (n = 9,928) were identified during 1987 through British pharmacists and pharmacy records. For comparison, an age-matched sample of cimetidine nonusers was chosen from the practices of the physicians who had prescribed cimetidine. One year later, the physicians' records of both groups were reviewed to determine the patients' status. (The results and limitations of this particular comparison are described later; see example on p. 117). By way of contrast, the *retrospective* approach was employed by O'Meara et al. (2001) to determine whether postmenopausal hormone therapy taken

---

[1] For therapies whose influence on a suspected adverse effect is believed to be very rapid, it is possible to compare the experience of persons who receive the therapy soon after it is given with their own experience at other times. The means by which this can be done has been described by Maclure (1991). Farrington et al. (1995) and Murphy et al. (2001) employed the approach to evaluate adverse effects following the administration of specific childhood vaccines.

by women who were clinically disease-free after initial breast cancer treatment had an adverse impact on the risk of cancer recurrence and mortality. Using cancer registry records, the investigators were able to identify female members of a prepaid health care plan who had been diagnosed with breast cancer during the period 1977–1994. From the pharmacy records of that same plan, women who had been prescribed estrogen hormones (with or without a progestogen) were enumerated from this cohort. Each of the 174 of these women who were also clinically disease free at the time of hormone initiation was matched to 4 other women with breast cancer. The latter were selected so as to be similar to their "index" case in terms of age, stage, and year of diagnosis, and they also were disease free as of the date the index cases' hormone use began. Medical records and cancer registry data were used to monitor recurrences and mortality in both the hormone users and hormone nonusers.

The issues governing the design, conduct, and analysis of cohort studies that evaluate unintended effects of therapy are in many ways similar to those of cohort studies that evaluate other exposures (e.g., occupational, environmental, dietary). The elaboration of these issues is best left to works on epidemiology per se. Nonetheless, there are several aspects of cohort studies of unintended effects that call for particular emphasis.

Identification and Characterization of Patients Who Receive a Given Therapy

Many adverse effects that occur soon (minutes to days) after administration of therapy can be identified by monitoring patients during a hospital stay (Miller, 1973). All therapies are recorded, and the patients' records are monitored for the occurrence of one or more of a large number of specified events (e.g., convulsions, electrocardiographic or electrolyte changes). The rates of each of these events in recipients and nonrecipients of various therapies are systematically compared.

There is a certain efficiency in in-hospital surveillance for adverse effects: large numbers of drugs and other therapeutic measures are prescribed in hospitals, and patients can be followed with relatively little expense by means of their charts. Still, an immense number of patients must be evaluated to adequately monitor drugs that are prescribed with low frequency in such a setting or to detect adverse effects that occur with low frequency. For example, in a surveillance program conducted in 1,669 pediatric inpatients, only 6 drugs (apart from oxygen, vitamins, and intravenous fluids) were administered to more than 200 children (Mitchell et al., 1979). Only 2 outcomes, fever and anemia, occurred in more than 100 children, and of course, in most instances these did not result from the use of a drug.

If treatment and illness data are retrievable on large numbers of outpatients, then this information can be used to assess adverse short-term treatment effects as well.

Example: In a study of possible drug etiologies of serum sickness, Heckbert et al. (1990) used the computerized records of the Harvard Community Health Plan to identify all children to whom cefaclor had been prescribed at any time during the period 1974–1986, along with a random sample of children given amoxicillin (total n = 3,487). During the 20-day period following the initiation of each course (there could be multiple courses) of either of these antibiotics, coded diagnoses of serum sickness, erythema multiforme, arthritis, or arthralgia were sought. The full medical records of all 40 children with these conditions were reviewed using standard criteria, resulting in confirmed diagnosis of serum sickness in 12 instances. Five of these cases had taken cefaclor and one had taken amoxicillin, corresponding to a nineteenfold greater incidence in the cefalor group.

To discover adverse effects that do not occur until weeks or years after therapy has been initiated, investigators must consider the experience of patients outside the hospital setting. Large numbers of persons (tens to hundreds of thousands) who have had drugs prescribed to them have been identified through computerized pharmacy records in prepaid health care plans in the United States (Friedman, 1978; Jick et al., 1981), in England through a central pricing authority (Skegg and Doll, 1981), and through government-run health care financing programs that cover whole populations (e.g., that of the Canadian province of Saskatchewan [Strand and West, 1989]) or subpopulations (e.g., medically indigent persons in the United States [Ray and Griffin, 1989; Gerstman et al., 1990a]). Also, it has become possible to identify drug prescriptions for individual patients from computerized records of a large number of general practitioners in the United Kingdom (Lis and Mann, 1995; Jick et al., 1991).

Nature of the Comparison Group

In theory, there are 2 options for comparison groups. Subjects can be drawn from persons who have the condition for which the treatment is given but who have not themselves been treated or who have been treated in a different manner. Or the comparison group can be drawn from the population of untreated persons in general, irrespective of whether they have the condition that leads to the particular therapy. What considerations guide the choice between these alternatives?

Ideally, *the comparison group should consist of untreated persons whose underlying risk (i.e., risk in the absence of the therapy) of the symptom/sign/ illness being investigated as a possible adverse effect is the same as that of the group that receives the therapy.* Persons who have the same conditions as those being treated but who themselves receive different (or no) therapy would seem to correspond most closely to the ideal, for then any associations found cannot be ascribed to the condition itself. For example, a greatly increased risk of acute leukemia was observed in cohort studies of alkylating agent therapy for ovarian cancer (Reimer et al., 1977) and of "intensive chemotherapy" (nitrogen mustard, procarbazine, prednisone, and either vincristine or vinblastine) for Hodgkin's disease (Boivin and Hutchinson, 1981). In both studies, the increase was apparent relative not only to incidence rates in the population as a whole but also to rates in patients with these neoplasms who did not receive the therapies. Thus one could rule out the possibility that the excess risk of leukemia was due solely to a predisposition to leukemia among persons with ovarian cancer or Hodgkin's disease.

In many situations, there is no ill-but-untreated group readily available for comparison. For example, in attempting to evaluate the long-term toxicity to DES exposure during pregnancy, it may prove difficult to identify a cohort of women who were pregnant during the 1950s, who were not given the drug, and who had the same indication for use (e.g., threatened spontaneous abortion) as did the DES-exposed group. Similarly, to evaluate the influence of neuroleptic agents on the incidence of breast cancer (these drugs stimulate prolactin secretion, which, in rodents, plays an etiologic role in mammary cancer), one may be hard pressed to identify women with comparable psychologic impairment at a corresponding point in time to whom these agents were not given.

If an illness itself is not associated with the occurrence of a particular adverse event, the use of persons who do not have the illness for which treatment was instituted has the potential to provide a valid result. Fortunately, this is usually the case. For example, apart from its necessitating the use of penicillin, pneumococcal pneumonia is unrelated to anaphylaxis or to the development of other allergic manifestations. Thus a valid measure of the role of penicillin in producing these allergic manifestations could be obtained by comparing their incidence in persons given penicillin with that in persons not given penicillin, irrespective of the pneumonia status of the latter group. In the same way, potential miscarriage or other reasons for prescribing DES during pregnancy probably are not themselves related to the development of vaginal adenosis in female offspring. Thus the daughters of women who did not take DES, whether or not the women were at increased risk of spontaneous abortion during pregnancy, are an appropriate group for comparison with daughters of DES-exposed women when evaluating vaginal adenosis and other possible adverse effects.

Nonetheless, there will be situations in which the lack of an ill-but-untreated group for comparison will render the results of the study uninterpretable: that is, it will prove impossible to separate the influence of the therapy in producing the suspected adverse effect from the influence of the illness for which the therapy was given.

Example: In the study mentioned previously, mortality among cimetidine users was compared with that among other (nonuser) patients in general, not specifically with mortality in persons with gastric acid-related disease who did not use cimetidine (Colin-Jones et al., 1983). This choice led to considerable ambiguity when the investigators attempted to interpret the initial results of the study:

Cause of death	Cumulative mortality (per 10,000) in first follow-up year	
	Cimetidine	Nonuser
All	377.7	211.7
Malignant neoplasm[a]		
Esophagus	7.1	1.1
Stomach	31.2	3.2
Bronchus and lung	18.1	11.8

[a] Patients who died of cancer that had been diagnosed prior to initiation of cimetidine therapy are excluded.

The investigators sought to eliminate a major bias that would have resulted from the preferential prescription of cimetidine to persons already diagnosed with a symptom-producing tumor of the upper gastrointestinal tract. Nonetheless, even after persons with these known antecedent conditions were excluded from the analysis, a large excess mortality for some of the same diseases (e.g., cancers of the esophagus, stomach, and lung) remained. Although these deaths could have been due to an effect of cimetidine, it is far more likely that they were the result of a not-yet-diagnosed disease process that led to the use of the drug. In the absence of a comparison group with symptoms similar to those of the patients given cimetidine, it is virtually impossible to discern any true effect of this drug on short-term mortality. Cognizant of the results of the preceding study, subsequent investigators of a possible longer term influence of cimetidine and other H_2 antagonists on the occurrence of stomach cancer (Schumacher et al., 1990) and adenocarcinoma of the esophagus (Chow et al., 1995) disregarded in their analyses cancer cases diagnosed within 1–2 years of the onset of therapy.

The study of Schumacher et al. (1990) is instructive for yet another strategy to distinguish a possible untoward effect of a drug from the indication that predisposed to its use. The authors observed that 5 of 99 persons (5.1%) with gastric cancer had begun to use cimetidine on a regular basis at least 2 years prior to diagnosis. Only 9 of 365 controls (2.5%) had done so. However, a similar difference was present for antacid use—among nonusers of cimetidine, 16.0% of cases versus 9.0% of controls had begun to take an antacid more than 2 years earlier and had continued to do so. Because it is unlikely that both cimetidine and antacid use can give rise to gastric cancer, it appears instead that an early stage of the cancer or the presence of a predisposing gastric lesion gave rise to both therapies.

Example: The patients of 20 British general practitioners were characterized regarding the use of drugs and subsequent illness events during
the period 1974–1976 (Skegg and Doll, 1981). Those who were prescribed dioctyl sodium sulfosuccinate, a fecal softening agent, were
found to have a higher incidence of chronic skin ulcers than other
patients of the same age and sex. Because those who did and did not
receive the agent were probably not comparable for the presence of
physical immobility—an important indication for fecal softening that
also strongly predicts the development of skin ulcers—the interpretation of the observed association is unclear.

Example: In the study by Skegg and Doll (1981), strong associations
were found between kaolin (a constituent of antidiarrheal preparations)
and rectal cancer and between the anticonvulsant phenytoin and brain
tumors. As the authors point out, almost certainly neither association
represented an adverse drug effect, but rather the use of the drug for
early symptoms of the underlying malignancy.

Ascertainment of the Potential Unintended Effects

Several methods of follow-up have been used to identify possible unintended effects of therapy over an extended period of time, including physician checklists and tumor registry data (Friedman, 1978; Selby et al., 1989),
computerized hospital discharge diagnoses (Jick et al., 1981; Smalley et al.,
1995), and a population-based morbidity and mortality reporting system
(Skegg and Doll, 1981). Whatever the means of the follow-up, the recognition of a manifestation that could represent an adverse effect should be made
equally well whether or not a patient has received the therapy under study.
There are 2 ways of attempting to achieve such equal recognition: (a) ascertainment with knowledge of exposure status withheld and (b) enumeration of
unambiguous criteria for the presence of the effect to be applied uniformly in
treated and untreated individuals. The first of these, "blind" ascertainment,
is rarely employed in nonrandomized studies of therapeutic safety because
nearly always such studies must rely on physicians to document or diagnose
the effect in their patients. Thus, even if the investigator assembles the data
without knowledge of treatment status, the data he or she is assembling may
incorporate a "detection" bias on the part of the patient's physician(s).

Thus, more commonly, cohort studies attempt to equalize ascertainment
using the second approach, standard criteria. Although this may be difficult
or impossible for potential adverse effects that often go undetected or un-
recorded (e.g., thrombophlebitis, gynecomastia), in many instances standard
criteria are easily applied and pose few or no problems in interpretation,
even when the standards are not very rigorous. For example, 17 cases of
non-Hodgkin's lymphoma were detected among 6,297 recipients of renal
transplants identified through an international transplant registry, whereas
only 0.5 cases would have been expected on the basis of incidence rates in

the general population (Hoover and Fraumeni, 1973). No attempt was made to standardize the criteria used to determine the presence of non-Hodgkin's lymphoma; the registry covered patients in 30 countries. Still, the association is almost certainly a real one, in part because of its magnitude but also because of the relatively similar criteria that would have been used between these patients and the comparison populations for the diagnosis of non-Hodgkin's lymphoma. (The issue of ascertainment in the follow-up for neoplasia in renal transplant recipients is, of course, distinct from the issue discussed earlier: that is, the separation of the influence of the underlying renal disease. Studies directed at distinguishing between these possibilities—cohort studies of persons with renal failure who did not receive a transplant—are not in full agreement, but it seems clear that whatever excess risk of non-Hodgkin's lymphoma might be present in such patients is considerably smaller than that which exists in the transplant recipients.)

It is important to recognize those situations in which the use of strict criteria in categorizing health outcomes is necessary in order for the study to have validity:

> *Example:* In late 1978, investigators in the Ohio Department of Health tried to quantify the association between vaccination against A/New Jersey influenza virus (swine flu) and the occurrence of the Guillain-Barre syndrome (GBS) (Marks and Halpin, 1980). Through Health Department records they were able to enumerate the approximately 2.2 million vaccinated persons. To ascertain cases of GBS, they queried neurologists in the state for cases diagnosed during and shortly after the time the vaccination program was taking place. The investigators were concerned that there might have been selective overascertainment of GBS patients who had been vaccinated, because (a) the diagnosis of GBS is not always clear-cut and (b) the ascertainment of cases took place during a period in which there was a considerable public speculation as to the presence of a swine flu-GBS link. Such speculation conceivably could have influenced neurologists to take account of vaccination status when considering a diagnosis of GBS. Thus the investigators required that, in order for a case to be accepted into the study, there must have been evidence of lower motor neuron weakness of acute onset. Patients given a diagnosis of GBS without such weakness were excluded. In addition, vaccinated and nonvaccinated cases were compared in terms of severity—if a diagnostic bias were present, the vaccinated cases would be expected to have been less severe on average—and no difference was found. Because of these measures, the four- to fivefold increased rate of GBS observed in vaccine recipients could be more readily interpreted as being attributable to the influence of the vaccine itself than to selective diagnostic error.

Some health events of interest are not recorded in a consistent way in the records available to those investigating potential adverse effects. For example, in one study (Gerstman et al., 1990b) an inpatient diagnosis of pulmonary embolism or venous thrombosis in 15- to 44-year old women was confirmed by expert record review as at least "probable" deep venous thrombosis in only 42% of instances. In such a circumstance, if detailed record review is not feasible, it may be possible to achieve a greater degree of specificity by augmenting diagnoses with data on medication prescribed in response to those diagnoses. In the previous example, 65% of women who had diagnoses of pulmonary embolism/venous thrombosis and had been prescribed an anticoagulant as outpatients were deemed on record review to have probably sustained deep venous thrombosis. Routine diagnoses of some conditions (e.g., depression) might be of low sensitivity. Thus several studies (Avorn et al., 1986; Thiessen et al., 1990) of possible associations between antihypertensive therapy and depression identified potential cases during follow-up solely through the receipt of a prescription for an antidepressant.

The incidence of some unintended consequences of a therapy varies with time since that therapy was administered. For example, mortality can be a complication of thoracic or abdominal surgery, but an increased risk of death may be present only during or soon after the operation. The use of medications containing phenylpropanolamine is hypothesized to predispose to cerebral hemorrhage, but largely or entirely in the first few hours or days after use has begun (Kernan et al., 2000). In contrast, whereas unopposed estrogen use by postmenopausal women almost certainly causes endometrial carcinoma, it appears to do so only after at least 1–2 years of use (Herrinton and Weiss, 1993).

In a cohort study of potential unintended health consequences of a treatment, the period of follow-up ideally should encompass the full range of intervals across which there may be variation in the presence (or size) of an altered risk. Thus a study of the unintended consequences of postmenopausal estrogen use ideally would monitor the health of women beginning at the time they are first prescribed this therapy, to identify a potential increase in risk of myocardial infarction or venous thromboembolism that may be present only at the outset of therapy. And that monitoring would continue for an extended period so that late effects, such as an increased risk of endometrial or breast cancer, could be identified as well. In practice, some studies may focus on the experience of persons relatively soon after therapy has begun and others on the long-term consequences, the overall impact of the therapy being judged by aggregating the results of the 2 types of study. The enumeration of a large enough number of persons beginning treatment to enable the detection of an altered risk of important, yet uncommon, adverse events can be challenging. Ray (2003) has discussed various approaches to accomplishing this.

Case-Control Studies

A case-control study evaluating therapeutic safety starts by identifying as "cases" persons who have developed a particular symptom, sign, or illness. It then identifies "controls," generally persons without the symptom, sign, or illness who are otherwise comparable to cases. In both groups it ascertains the proportion in whom the therapy under investigation has been received. To the extent that this proportion is increased among cases relative to controls, there is support for the contention that the symptom, sign, or illness represents an adverse effect of the therapy.

Are Case-Control Studies Really Necessary?

To many nonepidemiologists there is something unaesthetic about case-control studies. After all, why look for possible adverse effects in this backward sort of way? The answer is that for some adverse effects—those that are uncommon even in persons who received the therapies that produced them—there are no practical alternative means of identifying them. And, even though rare, some adverse effects are serious enough that knowledge of their presence can have a strong bearing on the decision to administer the therapy in question.

Earlier in this chapter we saw that randomized trials of DES during pregnancy failed to uncover the association with vaginal adenocarcinoma in the female children. Even after several hundred of the girls born to women who participated in these studies were located and examined 15 to 20 years later, no cases were found in either the DES-exposed or the comparison group (Bibbo et al., 1977; Beral and Colwell, 1981). These negative results can be attributed to the fact that vaginal adenocarcinoma is a rare enough condition, even in DES-exposed girls, that a true association with DES exposure could be missed in a group of this size. The same problem can plague a cohort study. For example, Lanier et al. (1973) monitored the incidence of cancer through the teenage years in 804 DES-exposed girls and also failed to find a case of vaginal adenocarcinoma.

It was through case-control studies that the association between in utero DES exposure and vaginal adenocarcinoma was identified. In the first study of this subject, for example, 7 of 8 cases had been exposed to DES, whereas fewer than 1 in 8 would have been expected based on the frequency in controls (Herbst et al., 1971). It was largely because of these data and those documenting the severity of this cancer that the Food and Drug Administration withdrew approval for the use of DES during pregnancy. This action was taken despite the fact that only a very small fraction of DES-exposed girls will suffer this adverse effect.

Obtaining a Valid Case-Control Comparison

In a case-control study that evaluates the safety of therapy, the function of a control group is to estimate the frequency with which a particular therapy would have been administered to persons who have developed the suspected adverse effect if the therapy itself played no causal role. Thus an ideal control group is one that consists of individuals:

(a) who are identical to the cases with respect to the distribution of all characteristics that (i) influence the likelihood of receiving the therapy and (ii) on their own also are related to the occurrence of the symptom, sign, or illness under study or to its recognition; and

(b) in whom a history of having received the therapy can be measured in a manner that is identical in accuracy to that used for cases.

There is no one way of defining controls that is best for every study. The choice is influenced largely by (a) the source from which the cases have been identified, (b) the influence of the treatment on the tendency to diagnose the suspected adverse event, (c) the relationship of the condition(s) for which the therapy is administered to the occurrence of this event, and (d) the kind of information on treatment history that can be obtained.

Source of Cases: Population-Based or Not?   When an investigator is able to identify all cases arising from a defined group of individuals, he or she generally chooses as controls a sample from other members of the defined group.[2] For example, some studies that have explored the possibility that postmenopausal hormone therapy might alter a user's risk of breast cancer (Chen et al., 2002; Ross et al., 1980; Schairer et al., 2000; Stanford et al., 1995) identified cases within defined populations: members of a prepaid health care plan, residents of a retirement community, enrollees for longitudinal monitoring at cancer detection clinics, and residents of a metropolitan county. Controls were, respectively, a sample of other women in the health care plan, other residents of the retirement community, other women undergoing screening, and other residents of the county. These choices allowed each study to achieve some degree of comparability among cases and controls with respect to a wide range of demographic characteristics that relate both to hormone use and to incidence of breast cancer. Also, this comparability could be achieved without having to sacrifice comparability of ascertainment of prior hormone use (see the following).

In many instances, however, the cases available for study do not relate to any defined population. Commonly, cases are chosen from persons who have selected a certain provider and/or institution for their care. In such instances, it is usually valid (and convenient) to select controls who are similar to the cases with respect to choice of health care provider/institution, excluding those who have conditions believed to be related to the treatment

[2] Strictly speaking, to enable the control group's experience to provide the most accurate estimate of the frequency with which a therapy has been administered in that population, persons who develop the symptom/sign/illness should be included as "controls" in proportion to their numbers in that population (Greenland and Thomas, 1982). This refinement, although appropriate, is seldom implemented. Its omission introduces virtually no bias until a high proportion—say, more than 20%—of treated individuals develops the adverse effect. (In such a situation, it is likely that a cohort study would be done instead.)

under study. So, when Kelsey et al. (1981) examined the possibility of an estrogen-breast cancer relationship by studying cancer cases from 3 Connecticut hospitals, controls were chosen from those admitted to inpatient surgical services at those same hospitals. Excluded as potential controls, however, were women who were gynecology patients, as it was felt that a number of them would have conditions that resulted from estrogen use (e.g., endometrial hyperplasia and carcinoma). The hope was that the remainder of the women admitted for surgery reflected closely the patterns of estrogen use in a hypothetical population whose members, if they were to have developed breast cancer, would have sought care in 1 of the 3 study hospitals.

> *Example:* In order to assess possible drug etiologies of acute severe cutaneous disorders (such as Stevens-Johnson syndrome and toxic epidermal necrolysis), a multicenter case-control study was initiated (Kelly et al., 1995). Persons admitted with one of these rare conditions were identified in burn and intensive care units and in dermatology and pediatric wards in institutions in France, Germany, Italy, and Portugal. They (or their parents) were queried regarding medications taken in the 4 weeks prior to the development of the first symptom of their illness. Because there was no practical way of sampling directly from the population from which the cases arose, controls were obtained instead from persons admitted to those same institutions with an acute condition, such as an infection, fracture, or an abdominal emergency. Their use of medications in the 4 weeks prior to the onset of illness or injury was sought in a manner identical to that for the cases.

What can be learned from studies that select as cases only those patients who have received the therapy in question? The British Committee on Safety of Medicines based a study on the reports they received of women who sustained a cardiovascular "event" who had been using oral contraceptives. In another study, in the United States, an attempt was made to identify users of oral contraceptives who developed endometrial cancer prior to 40 years of age. Both studies have produced important data on the safety of oral contraceptives, but only because there was heterogeneity within the type of therapy (i.e., oral contraceptives of different formulations) and because there were some data external to the study to help gauge the way in which the heterogeneity would have been expected to manifest itself (i.e., some data on the relative frequency of use of the various oral contraceptive preparations). Thus, when Meade et al. (1980) analyzed the type of oral contraceptive used by the British women who were reported as having sustained a cardiovascular event, they found an overrepresentation of preparations with high progestogen levels relative to that expected on the basis of sales by British pharmacists. In the American women who had taken oral contraceptives and who developed endometrial cancer, 19 of 30 had taken Oracon (Silverberg et al., 1977), a far higher proportion than would have been anticipated on the basis of Oracon's share of the U.S. oral contraceptive market.

It must be remembered that these studies of heterogeneity among treated persons provide evidence only of the relative safety of one preparation vis-à-vis another. For example, Oracon users could be overrepresented among endometrial cancer patients who used oral contraceptives because either Oracon predisposes the user to the disease or the use of other preparations reduces the incidence of the disease. The only way to distinguish between these possibilities is to do the more conventional type of case-control study in which women with and without the cancer (selected without regard to the use of the pill) are compared regarding their prior use of oral contraceptives. Indeed, when this was done, both an excess of Oracon use and a deficit of use of other oral contraceptives were found in women with endometrial cancer (Weiss and Sayvetz, 1980).

Influence of Treatment on Detection of the Suspected Adverse Effect   The recognition by physicians of signs, symptoms, and illnesses is imperfect, and sometimes it is influenced by the patient's previous therapy history. For instance, it has been suggested that physicians are more likely to perform diagnostic tests for endometrial cancer in women who use estrogens than in other women (Horwitz and Feinstein, 1978). If this is true, and if some cases of endometrial cancer never become sufficiently symptomatic to elicit diagnostic activity, then a spurious (or spuriously large) association between estrogen use and endometrial cancer could arise.

The same sort of bias might be present when trying to determine whether estrogen use predisposes patients to gallstone disease. Many women who have gallstones never have them diagnosed (Gracie and Ransohoff, 1982). Compared with such women, those in whom the diagnosis is made might be expected, on the average, to see a physician on a regular basis and to seek active medical intervention (e.g., diagnostic testing and surgery) for symptoms. These are also characteristics that, on the average, estrogen users might be expected to have to a greater extent than nonusers. Thus, if estrogen-use histories were compared between women diagnosed as having (or being treated surgically for) gallstones and a "typical" control group, falsely large estimates of an association could be obtained.

Concerns such as these led one group of investigators, when conducting a case-control study of endometrial cancer, to pick a control group that underwent the same degree of diagnostic evaluation as did the cases; they chose women without endometrial cancer who underwent uterine dilation and curettage (D&C) or endometrial biopsy (Horwitz and Feinstein, 1978). Their results, in contrast to those of nearly all other studies of the subject (in which controls were not required to have undergone these diagnostic tests), showed virtually no association between estrogen use and endometrial cancer; there were nearly identical patterns of estrogen use in cases and controls. Unfortunately, in the process of eliminating one source of bias (that relating to differential cancer detection in users and nonusers), their design created another: Those postmenopausal women who undergo a D&C or endometrial biopsy but who do not have endometrial cancer generally have a bleeding disorder caused by a hyperplastic process in the endometrium. A common cause of endometrial hyperplasia is estrogen use, and so a history of estrogen use among such women would be very common. Using them as controls could (and did) nullify any true association of endometrial cancer with estrogen use.

Despite the fact that this strategy (of choosing controls from patients undergoing the diagnostic test(s) for the suspected adverse effect) did not "work" for endometrial cancer, there probably are some situations in which its use has merit. One might be the study of a possible estrogen-gallstone disease association, for there is no reason to believe that an association exists between estrogen use and the presence of symptoms that led to a negative cholecystogram or ultrasound test.

When controls are chosen from persons who have not been evaluated for the suspected adverse effect, another concern is often expressed: To the extent that there are cases mixed into this group, will not the resulting contamination lead to the case and control groups being artificially similar with respect to a history of having received the therapy? Such concern will be unwarranted any time the prevalence of the suspected adverse effect is low (which is most of the time), for the inclusion of an occasional occult case in a large group of noncases will have only a small impact on the results.

Influence of the Condition for Which the Therapy Is Administered on the Occurrence of the Symptom, Sign, or Illness   Controls should be matched to cases with regard to indication for treatment only if the indication itself predisposes to the occurrence of the condition that defines the case group or predisposes to its recognition. Such matching is seldom needed—rarely are both the condition being treated and the treatment given under suspicion as possibly causing the same adverse effect. Nonetheless, there are instances in which failure to match (or otherwise control) for "indication" leads to an ambiguous result. For example, the use of "minor" tranquilizers among persons injured in vehicular accidents was compared with that among persons chosen at random from the population (Skegg et al., 1979). During the 3-month period preceding the injury, cases were 5 times more likely than controls to have been prescribed one of these agents. Although this result could indicate an adverse effect of minor tranquilizers, it could as well be interpreted to indicate an underlying tendency for persons to whom these drugs are prescribed to sustain a vehicular injury. Because the investigators were unable to match on, and had no data available to control for, the "need" for these tranquilizers, both interpretations remain viable.

The Kind of Information on Treatment History That Can Be Obtained   No matter how comparable a control and a case are in other respects, differences between them in the ability to ascertain a history of therapy will distort the results of a study and possibly invalidate it altogether. Ideally, then, such ascertainment should be identical for cases and controls, with no opportunity for bias based on awareness of subsequent events. This ideal sometimes can be met when treatment records are compiled prior to the occurrence of the suspected adverse effects. For example, in a study of breast cancer by Hoover et al. (1981), outpatient records of women prior to other diagnosis (and prior to a corresponding date for controls) were reviewed for possible hormone and other drug exposures. This review was done without knowledge of the case/control status of the women whose records were being reviewed. In another case-control study that ascertained drug use through review of medical records, this one on renal cell cancer (Weinmann et al., 1994), it was not practical to blind those persons conducting the review to the subjects' status as a case or control. However, to minimize potential bias resulting from there being extensive recent chart information on the cases—due to their hospitalization for and treatment of the cancer—but not necessarily on the controls, the investigators restricted the record review to a time period ending 3 months prior to the development of the symptoms that led to diagnosis (and the corresponding interval for controls). Clearly, this latter strategy would not be appropriate when studying potential unintended medication effects with a relatively rapid induction period.

Objective information on drugs prescribed for cases and controls also can be obtained from computerized records of some payers for health care (e.g., Medicaid) or from some providers (e.g., certain prepaid health care plans). The presence of such computerized records on large populations can lead to a statistically powerful assessment of the impact of even uncommonly used medications.

Example: Juurlink et al. (2003) conducted a case-control study among the 1.5 million residents of the province of Ontario who were 65 years and older. Through the records of the Ontario Drug Benefit Program, they identified 523 persons who were being prescribed an angiotensin-converting enzyme (ACE) inhibitor and who, while they were on this drug, developed hyperkalemia (as identified in the Canadian Institute for Health Information Discharge Database). For these 523 "cases" and 25,807 controls—persons receiving an ACE inhibitor who were not diagnosed with hyperkalemia, matched to the cases on age, sex, and the presence or absence of renal disease—they ascertained (again through the computerized records of the Drug Benefit Program) use of a potassium-sparing diuretic during the preceding week. In 8.2% of the cases, but in only 0.3% of the controls, a potassium-sparing drug had been prescribed (adjusted relative risk = 20.3). In the absence of computerized information on both prescription drugs and health outcomes on a large population, it is unlikely that this striking drug-drug interaction could have been documented.

Prescribing a pharmaceutical agent, of course, does not guarantee that it will be taken. For studies of potential long-term effects of medication use ascertained by means of computerized pharmacy records, some investigators (e.g., Dublin et al. [2002] in a study of ovarian cancer in relation to use of antidepressants and benzodiazepines) have in their analyses limited "users" to persons who filled at least 2 prescriptions for a given medication. Case-control studies based on computerized pharmacy data also may be limited by a person's relatively short participation in a particular health care plan or by the length of time the computerized data are available. The longer the duration of medication use needed to produce an altered risk of an unintended outcome, or the longer the interval between the time that use begins and the time the outcome occurs, the less useful computerized pharmacy data are in addressing the question. Records of therapy, particularly drug therapy administered some years earlier, may not be easy to assemble and, indeed, may not be available. Therefore, in many case-control studies of therapeutic safety, it is necessary to rely on the memory of the subject. For many forms of therapy, particularly surgical procedures or drugs taken for extended periods of time, memory can be trusted to be both sensitive and specific. For instance, women's statements of prior hysterectomy/oophorectomy and long-term menopausal estrogen use have been evaluated against medical records and found to be quite accurate (Jick et al., 1980; Brinton et al., 1981).

As might be expected, a subject's memory will be not so accurate for short-term drug therapy, particularly if it occurred in the not-so-recent past. Yet some of these short-term exposures could be associated with adverse drug effects. Drug therapy of even a few day's duration in pregnancy, for example (particularly in the first trimester), could be associated with abnormalities in the children. However, the ability of mothers of abnormal and normal newborns to remember events of early pregnancy may vary considerably, and data from comparisons of 2 groups such as these must be interpreted with some caution. One approach to minimizing this type of recall bias has been to compare drugs taken by mothers of children with a particular type of abnormality (or collection of related abnormalities) with those taken by mothers of children with all *other* abnormalities. Presumably, the recall by women in the 2 groups would be comparable. Unless the drug were associated with a large number of different abnormalities, such a comparison should offer a relatively unbiased evaluation of the drug's safety.

Example: In a case-control study of birth defects, women who had just delivered a child in one of several hospitals were interviewed (Rosenberg et al., 1983). The use of diazepam during the first trimester of pregnancy was equally common in mothers of children with isolated cleft palate or cleft lip (with or without cleft palate) as in the combined group of mothers of children with any other malformation. Thus, assuming that diazepam does not produce a broad range of birth defects, the development of oral clefts during fetal life does not appear to be related to exposure to this drug.

Incorporating Results of Case-Control Studies into the Decision-Making Process

When trying to arrive at a decision regarding the use of a therapy, it is necessary to balance rates (and severity) of any adverse effects against rates (and severity) of progression or complications of the condition for which the therapy is administered. So, even if it is conceded that case-control studies are capable of identifying the *existence* of an adverse effect, the important question of its *frequency* following treatment is left unresolved.

Fortunately, once a case-control study has indicated an association of therapy with an unintended effect and the effect is judged to be a result of therapy, it is usually possible to derive a reasonable estimate of the frequency with which the effect occurs. This estimate is obtained in 2 steps. First, it is necessary to calculate the incidence of the unintended effect in persons given the treatment in question relative to that in other persons. Although the case-control study measures only the frequency with which the *treatment* has been administered, the relative incidence of the adverse *effect* can be approximated by means of the odds ratio, as illustrated in Table 6.1. In the example, the data indicate a greater frequency of oral contraceptive use among young women who died of a myocardial infarction than among controls, the incidence in users estimated as being 2.8 times that in nonusers.

Table 6.1. Method of Estimating Relative Incidence of an Adverse Effect from Results of a Case-Control Study

General		Unintended effect		Example		Myocardial infarction[a]	
		Present	Absent			Yes	No
Therapy administered	Yes	a	b	Current oral contraceptive	Yes	21	17
	No	c	d	use:	No	26	59
		$a + c$	$b + d$			47	76

Odds of exposure in cases = a/c Odds of exposure in cases = 21/26
Odds of exposure in controls = b/d Odds of exposure in controls = 17/59

Odds ratio $\cong$ relative incidence   Odds ratio $\cong$ relative incidence

$$= \frac{a/c}{b/d} = \frac{a \times d}{b \times c}$$ $$= \frac{21/26}{17/59} = \frac{21 \times 59}{26 \times 17} = 2.8$$

[a] Deaths in women aged 30–39 years (Mann and Inman, 1975).

The explanation as to why these frequencies of "exposure" can be manipulated to produce an estimate of relative incidence (often termed "relative risk") is contained in epidemiology textbooks (Koepsell and Weiss, 2003), as are the assumptions required for the estimate to be a valid one (principally, a cumulative incidence of the unintended effect in exposed persons of less than 20% to 25%).

The second step in estimating the incidence of an adverse effect involves multiplying the value obtained for relative incidence by the underlying rate of the effect in persons who have not received the therapy. The underlying rate can be obtained in one of several ways, often from published rates for populations in whom the therapy has not been used or in which the large majority of cases are not related to the therapy.

> *Example:* You look up the mortality rate from myocardial infarction in 30- to 39-year-old women during a period just before oral contraceptive use became widespread and find it to have been 1.9 per 100,000 per year. Thus the annual mortality rate from this cause in an oral contraceptive user would be expected to be about $2.8 \times 1.9/100,000/\text{year} = 5.4/100,000/\text{year}$.

What if you are not quite sure of the underlying rate you have identified? What if it might not quite be the one that prevails in your particular untreated population? Simply choose a range of plausible values for the rate and, over the whole of the range, calculate a rate of the unintended effect in treated persons. Incorporate each of the resulting rates, one at a time, into the weighing of risks and benefits of the therapy (e.g., through decision analysis). For many therapies, the decision regarding use will be the same across the plausible range of incidence rates.

Association between the Use of a Therapy and the Occurrence of an Unintended Event: When Does It Represent Causation?

There are several possible explanations for an association seen in nonrandomized studies between treatment and an unintended event, and only one of these is that the treatment caused the event. First, measurement error could be responsible: Perhaps discovery of the condition was incomplete but less so in patients who received the treatment. Second, the patient groups being evaluated for the occurrence of an unintended event (or, in a case-control study, for a history of having received the therapy) could be dissimilar regarding their underlying risk of the event, leading to an apparent association with therapy when none truly exists. Finally, the association could simply be due to chance: The experience of the particular sample of subjects in the study may not really reflect that of the larger group of individuals to whom the findings are to be generalized.

Now, the means of distinguishing between these possible explanations is to a large extent subjective, and thus it is by no means infallible. Fortunately, there are some guidelines that have served well in the past in trying to accomplish this task.

1. To what degree is the incidence of the unintended event increased in

persons receiving the therapy relative to that in other persons? The greater the relative incidence, the less likely it is that noncausal explanations could account for it.

What about using the P value for this purpose, that is, as a measure of the "strength" of an association? The P value is calculated for another important but narrower reason: It answers the question, What would be the likelihood of observing this degree of excess risk (or more) if there were no true association between therapy and the adverse event? In arriving at an answer, the P value takes into account not only the size of the association but also the number of subjects studied. For any given difference, a study with a large number of subjects will produce a smaller P value than will one with a small number. But, of course, the number of subjects enrolled in a study is controlled primarily by practical considerations and so must not be a factor when trying to assess the presence of a biological relationship.

Let's say that 7% of controls had been given drug X during the past year. It is far easier to attribute causality if 90% of cases had received drug X during that time than if 10% had received it, even if in both instances the case-control differences had been "statistically significant" to the same degree. In clinical epidemiologic studies, there almost always are too many sources of confounding and bias to be confident that the difference between 7% and 10% reflects the causal influence of drug X in producing the effect, no matter what the P value. A difference between 7% and 90%, however, similar to that seen in the example of DES and vaginal adenocarcinoma, is harder to fully account for by noncausal explanations.

2. Is it clear that the administration of the therapy has preceded the presence of the suspected unintended effect? For most observed associations between a therapy and an event, there is no ambiguity in the temporal relation. For example, chloramphenicol and clozapine unequivocally predate the aplastic anemia with which each is associated. But there are instances in which the design of the study that has documented an association has failed to clearly identify whether the therapy or the suspected unintended event came first. Earlier, we saw that an elevated mortality rate of gastrointestinal cancers soon after the initiation of cimetidine could not be interpreted, as it was all too likely that the association resulted from the action of clinically occult tumors producing symptoms that led to the use of this drug. As another example, Avorn et al. (1986) observed that Medicaid recipients who were prescribed beta blockers for hypertension during a 2-year period more commonly also received tricyclic antidepressants (a marker for clinical depression) during that period than did persons prescribed other antihypertensive agents. However, because the investigators did not determine which drug had been prescribed first (either in that 2-year period or earlier), the meaning of these results is unclear. To clarify the temporal sequence of events, subsequent studies have sought to compare the incidence only of new diagnoses of depression or initiation of antidepressive therapy between users of beta blockers and other persons (Bright and Everitt, 1992).

Investigators of a possible association between aspirin use and the development of Reye's syndrome had to contend with a possibly ambiguous temporal relation of drug and outcome, given that Reye's syndrome is usually preceded by a flu-like illness for which aspirin may be taken. Conceivably, the antecedent illness could represent the earliest phase of Reye's syndrome itself, and the observed high frequency of aspirin use in children with the disease could have occurred as a consequence of the illness rather than being a causal factor. The strategy most investigators adopted was a case-control study using, as controls, children without Reye's syndrome who had the same type and severity of antecedent illness as did the cases. To the extent that they were successful in doing this, the large observed difference in aspirin use between cases and controls could be interpreted as indicating a causal relation.

3. How plausible is the hypothesis that the association between therapy and event is a causal one, in terms of knowledge gained in other areas? The more credible the pharmacologic or physiologic explanations for such an association, the more we are inclined to accept the hypothesis that the association represents cause and effect. Thus the results of case-control studies showing differences in the prior use of postmenopausal estrogens by women with endometrial cancer and by controls were widely accepted as indicative of a causal connection, partly because the case-control differences in use were large but also because (a) prolonged exposure to elevated levels of endogenous estrogens was known to be associated with an increased risk of endometrial cancer; (b) the case-control difference was present only for "long" durations of estrogen use (i.e., several or more years); and (c) the rates of endometrial cancer in the population rapidly rose and fell in parallel with the level of the population's consumption of estrogens. This last observation made it particularly hard to accept the alternative hypothesis for the presence of the association, that is, that the conditions necessitating the use of estrogens (e.g., hot flashes) were risk factors for endometrial cancer even in the absence of estrogen use. It was implausible that the prevalence of these necessitating conditions was rising and falling over such a relatively short period of time.

Absolute "proof" that a therapy produces a particular unintended effect is *never* forthcoming. Causes are inferred, not observed, and inferences require subjective judgments that often differ among individuals. Yet it is necessary to attempt to draw inferences of cause and effect even from inevitably incomplete data, for the alternative is to make no inference at all, which would preclude taking preventive or therapeutic action.

Questions

6.1. In prelicensing randomized trials of rotavirus vaccines, there were a total of 5 cases of intussusception (a form of bowel obstruction) among 10,054 infants who received the vaccine (0.05%). Among 4,633 placebo recipients, there was but 1 case (0.02%). The observed difference in the cumulative incidence of 0.03% was easily compatible with there being no true excess risk associated with the vaccine ($p > 0.45$).

What is your principal reservation in concluding from these data that immunization against rotavirus is not related to an increased risk of intussusception?

6.2. In December 1989, cyclosporine replaced azathioprine as the drug with which physicians at Stanford University attempted to achieve immunosuppression in patients undergoing cardiac transplantation. They noted that in the 32 patients who received a transplant after that date and who survived for 1 year, the mean serum creatinine rose from a presurgery value of 1.3 to 2.1 mg/dl ($P = 0.01$). Other measures of glomerular filtration rate were also depressed after transplantation. What other patient group's experience should be reviewed for comparison to determine whether the administration of cyclosporine has an adverse effect on renal function?

6.3. There has been a widely held belief among physicians that the occurrence of psychiatric disorders in general, and depression in particular, is inordinately common in women who have undergone hysterectomy. To determine whether this association is indeed present, and to better delineate the possible causal role of the hysterectomy itself, a cohort study was conducted (Barker, 1968). Female residents of Dundee, Scotland, who had undergone hysterectomies during the years 1960–1964 were identified through hospital records. The large majority of these operations had been performed for nonmalignant conditions. For comparison, a sample of Dundee women who had had cholecystectomies during the same period were identified. Records of referrals to psychiatrists in that city were examined through 1966 (i.e., a minimum of 2 years of follow-up) to locate names of women in both cohorts.

In the first 2 years after surgery, 3.2% of the hysterectomy cohort had been referred to psychiatrists, in contrast to only 1.2% of the cholecystectomy cohort ($P = 0.01$ for the age-adjusted difference). The observed association was not attributable to the simultaneous removal of the ovaries of women in the hysterectomy group, as only 19% also had undergone oophorectomy and the incidence of referral for these women was similar to that of the hysterectomy group as a whole. Neither could the association be explained by a higher measured level of presurgical psychiatric morbidity in women undergoing hysterectomy, for prior to surgery their likelihood of referral had been nearly the same as that of women in the cholecystectomy group. Finally, by including women undergoing cholecystectomy for comparison, the author could exclude the possibility that surgical procedures in general were responsible for the increased psychiatric referral rate.

Nonetheless, despite the observed association and these strengths of the study design, you have an important reservation about concluding that hysterectomy predisposes patients to psychiatric morbidity. What is it?

6.4. Following the publication in the *New England Journal of Medicine* of the results of several case-control studies that examined the relationship of diazepam use during the first trimester of pregnancy to the occurrence of oral clefts in the offspring, 2 investigators wrote a letter to the editor (Shiono and Mills, 1984). They stated that "the problem with the [case-control] approach is that using normal controls might lead to underreporting of exposure, whereas using [other] malformed controls might result in diazepam-induced malformations in the control group. In either instance, an erroneous estimate of risk would result."

They provided data from a follow-up study that they said "avoids these pitfalls," in which the use of diazepam (and other drugs) was ascertained during an interview at the first prenatal visit.

First trimester exposure to diazepam	Oral cleft		
	Yes	No	Total
Yes	1	853	854
No	31	32,364	32,395

a. What was the risk of oral cleft in a child whose mother had used diazepam during the first trimester of pregnancy?

b. What was the risk relative to the risk in children who were not so exposed?

c. The data from the follow-up study that the investigators presented also have limitations, relative to those from case-control studies, in evaluating a potential diazepam—oral cleft association. What do you believe to be the main limitation?

6.5. On learning of several laboratory studies suggesting that cardiac glycosides inhibit tumor growth, 2 investigators decided to do a case-control study (Goldin and Safa, 1984). They reviewed the medical records of 69 patients who died in their hospital; in 21 patients, the cause of death was cancer. Only 1 of these patients had been treated previously with digitalis preparations, in contrast to 18 or 48 patients who died from other causes.

From these data, can you estimate the risk of death from cancer in persons who use digitalis preparations relative to the risk in other persons? If so, what is that relative risk? If not, why not?

What is the most likely reason that these results overstate the influence of digitalis preparations on the occurrence of death from cancer?

6.6. A case-control study of myocardial infarction in young women obtained the following results:

Number of risk factors	Type of risk factor	Cases (%)	Controls (%)
None	—	18.9	64.0
Only one	Oral contraceptive use	5.4	4.5
	Hyperlipidemia	5.4	0.5
	Cigarette smoking	16.2	16.5
	Hypertension	6.8	9.5
	Diabetes	1.4	0.0
Any two of the above	—	27.0	4.5
Three or more of the above	—	18.9	0.5
		100	100

A reviewer claimed that because the percentages of cases and controls were nearly identical (5.4% and 4.5%), these data indicated virtually no increased risk of myocardial infarction in users of oral contraceptives who had none of the other risk factors. Would you agree with this claim? If yes, why? If no, why not?

6.7. To determine whether drug regimens used for ovarian stimulation were associated with an altered risk of cancer, women in Victoria, Australia, who had undergone one or more in vitro fertilization (IVF) treatment cycles ($n = 5,564$) were compared with infertile women who had been referred for IVF but had not been treated ($n = 4,794$) (Venn et al., 1995). The interval between initial referral and the receipt of IVF varied from patient to patient and ranged from 0 to 3 years. Study participants who developed cancer were identified through records of a population-based cancer registry that serves the state of Victoria. The rates of cancer in the IVF and non-IVF women, following the initiation of IVF or registration with the IVF clinic, respectively, were adjusted for any differences between them regarding age and type of infertility.

To at least a small degree, this approach will overestimate the risk of cancer in infertile women who do not receive IVF and thus underestimate the relative risk of cancer associated with the receipt of IVF. Why?

Answers

6.1. Even though more than 14,000 infants were studied, intussusception is so uncommon that the observed 2.5-fold increase (0.0005/0.0002) is well within the bounds of chance given no true adverse influence of rotavirus immunization. The studies were not large enough, collectively, to reliably determine the presence of an association of this magnitude. The question was better addressed in a U.S. 19-state case-control study (Murphy et al., 2001) that enrolled 429 infants with intussusception. Although the relative risk estimated from the data gathered in the case-control study was similar to that observed collectively in the randomized trials—2.2 versus 2.5—the 95% confidence interval, in contrast, was quite narrow (1.5–3.3), and the P value was quite small (< 0.001).

6.2. The investigators faced the task of separating the effects of cyclosporine administration from other aspects of cardiac transplantation and its physiologic consequences as factors responsible for the deterioration in renal function. They sought to do this by examining renal function in a comparison cohort: cardiac transplant patients who underwent their surgery before cyclosporine therapy was instituted (i.e., before December 1980) (Myers et al., 1984). There were 47 such patients who survived at least 1 year; all had received another immunosuppressive agent, azathioprine. Their mean serum creatinine after the transplantation was, if anything, somewhat lower than it had been (1.0 vs. 1.3 mg/dl prior to surgery).

These results argue strongly that cyclosporine produces renal dysfunction, although it should not be forgotten that the following assumptions are being made: (a) there were no other changes in the care of heart transplant patients introduced at about the same time as cyclosporine that produce renal damage and (b) there have been no trends over time in the propensity of patients undergoing heart transplantation to develop renal damage.

6.3. The main limitation of this study lies in the insensitive nature of the measure of psychiatric morbidity (i.e., referral to a psychiatrist) and of possible bias resulting from the use of that measure. It is not that you believe the investigator to have been biased in ascertaining the occurrence of psychiatric referral among members of the 2 cohorts. Rather, you are concerned that (a) only a small percentage of women with psychiatric morbidity are referred to psychiatrists and (b) referral of an individual patient by her physician may be prompted by his or her belief that women are prone to suffer emotionally following a hysterectomy. Far more convincing would have been a study, otherwise designed as well as this one, that in a standardized and unbiased way obtained a direct measurement of psychiatric functioning (e.g., by personal interview) in the 2 groups of women.

6.4.a. Risk of oral cleft = 1/854 = 0.012

   b. Relative risk = $1/854 \div 31/32{,}364 = 1.22$

   c. This study has eliminated both potential "pitfalls" that it cites: There is no bias in the ascertainment of diazepam use relative to oral cleft occurrence, because knowledge of the presence or absence of the malformation occurred after the drug history was obtained; and the comparison group is not restricted to children with other conditions that could have been associated with diazepam exposure.

Unfortunately, it has replaced these limitations with another: It has the ability to reliably identify only a very large association between diazepam use and oral clefts. For example, even if the true incidence ratio had been 3.0, this study would have had only about a 45% chance of finding a significant difference (at the 5% level) in the occurrence of oral clefts between the offspring of diazepam users and nonusers. Note that in a study of more than 33,000 pregnancies, only 32 babies with clefts were available for study. A case-control study, whatever its problems may or may not be in this instance with respect to accurate ascertainment of diazepam use, could very likely achieve a larger sample of such cases, with a corresponding increase in power. The rarer the suspected adverse effect, the more a case-control study will be needed if its association with a given exposure is to be identified.

6.5. In a case-control study of death from cancer, it is possible to estimate the relative cancer mortality associated with use of a particular therapy by dividing the odds that cases have been exposed to digitalis by the odds that controls have been exposed:

Used digitalis	Patients with cancer	Patients dying of other causes (controls)
Yes	1	18
No	20	30

$$\text{Relative mortality} = \frac{1/20}{18/30} = 0.08$$

If this case-control comparison were valid (it is not; see the following), it would suggest that the cancer mortality of users of digitalis preparations is only 8% that of nonusers.

This study is flawed primarily by the nature of the comparison group. It is likely that a sizable proportion of the group chosen—persons who died of causes other than cancer—died of cardiovascular disease and thus would contain an inordinately high number of patients who had received digitalis preparations. Even if the use of digitalis among cancer patients were perfectly typical of the population as a whole (i.e., no true association), the use of this particular control group would lead to the finding of an apparent protective effect of these drugs. Indeed, when the digitalis-cancer association was investigated by means of more appropriate comparisons, a suggestion of a modest increase in risk was found (Friedman, 1984).

6.6. The possible association between the use of oral contraceptives and myocardial infarction in young women with no other measured risk factors must utilize the following data:

	Cases (%)	Controls (%)
Oral contraceptive use only	5.4	4.5
No risk factor	18.9	64.0

$$\text{Relative incidence} = \frac{5.4/18.9}{4.5/64.0} = 4.1$$

The results of this study suggest a fourfold increase in the risk of myocardial infarction among young women with no other risk factors in relation to the use of oral contraceptives. A comparison only of the percentages of cases and controls with no other risk factors who used oral contraceptives— a comparison that ignores the very different percentages of cases and controls with no risk factors at all—would lead to a mistaken conclusion.

6.7. Omitted from the authors' analysis was the person-time experience of IVF recipients that accrued between registration and the time of the first IVF stimulation. (If a cancer had been diagnosed during this period, it would have been counted as having occurred in a woman who had not undergone IVF.) By not including the months to years prior to the start of IVF in the calculation of cancer incidence in non-IVF women, the authors overestimated these rates, and so underestimated the relative rates in women who did receive IVF.

References

Avorn J, Everitt DE, Weiss S. Increased antidepressant use in patients prescribed ß-blockers. *JAMA* 1986;255:357–360.

Barker MG. Psychiatric illness after hysterectomy. *Br Med J* 1968;2:91–95.

Beral V, Colwell L. Randomized trial of high doses of stilboestrol and esthisterone therapy in pregnancy: Long-term follow-up of the children. *J Epidemiol Community Health* 1981;35:155–160.

Bernstein HN. Chloroquine ocular toxicity. *Surv Ophthalmol* 1967;12:415–417.

Bibbo M, Gill WB, Freidoon A, et al. Follow-up study of male and female offspring of DES-exposed mothers. *J Obstet Gynecol* 1977;49:1–8.

Boivin JF, Hutchison GB. Leukemia and other cancers after radiotherapy and chemotherapy for Hodgkin's disease. *J Nat Cancer Inst* 1981;67:751–760.

Bright RA, Everitt DE. ß-blockers and depression: Evidence against an association. *JAMA* 1992;267:1783–1787.

Brinton LA, Hoover RN, Szklo M, et al. Menopausal estrogen use and risk of breast cancer. *Cancer* 1981;47:2517–2522.

Chen C-L, Weiss NS, Newcomb P, et al. Hormone replacement therapy in relation to breast cancer. *JAMA* 2002;287:734–741.

Chow WH, Finkle WD, McLaughlin JK, et al. The relation of gastroesophageal reflux disease and its treatment to adenocarcinomas of the esophagus and gastric cardia. *JAMA* 1995:274:474–477.

Colin-Jones DG, Langman MJ, Lawson DH, et al. Postmarketing surveillance of the safety of cimetidine: 12 month mortality report. *Br Med J* 1983;286:1713–1716.

Dublin S, Rossing MA, Heckbert SR, et al. Risk of epithelial ovarian cancer in relation to use of antidepressants, benzodiazopines, and other centrally acting medications. *Cancer Causes Control* 2002;13:35–45.

Farrington P, Pugh S, Colville A, et al. A new method for active surveillance of adverse events from diphtheria/tetanus/pertussin and measles/mumps/rubella vaccines. *Lancet* 1995;345:567–569.

Friedman GD. Digitalis and breast cancer. *Lancet* 1984;2:875.

Friedman GD. Monitoring of drug effects in outpatients: Development of a program to detect carcinogenesis. In Ducrot H et al. (eds), *Computer Aid to Drug Therapy and to Drug Monitoring*. Amsterdam: North-Holland, 1978:55–62.

Gerstman BB, Lundin FE, Stadel BV, et al. A method of pharmacoepidemiologic analysis that uses computerized Medicaid. *J Clin Epidemiol* 1990a; 43:1387–1393.

Gerstman BB, Freiman JP, Hine LK. Use of subsequent anticoagulants to increase the predictive value of Medicaid deep venous thromboembolism diagnosis. *Epidemiol* 1990b;1:122–127.

Goldin AG, Safa AR. Digitalis and cancer. *Lancet* 1984;1:1134.

Gracie WA, Ransohoff DF. The natural history of silent gallstones: The innocent gallstone is not a myth. *N Engl J Med* 1982;307:798–800.

Greene MH, Boice JD, Greer BE, et al. Acute nonlymphocytic leukemia after therapy with alkylating agents for ovarian cancer: A study of five randomized clinical trials. *N Engl J Med* 1982;307:1416–1421.

Greenland S, Thomas DC. On the need for the rare disease assumption in case-control studies. *Am J Epidemiol* 1982;1116:547–553.

Heckbert SR, Stryker WS, Coltin KL, et al. Serum sickness in children after antibiotic exposure estimates of occurrence and morbidity in a health maintenance organization population. *Am J Epidemiol* 1990;132:336–342.

Herbst AL, Ulfelder H, Poskanzer DC. Adenocarcinoma of the vagina: Association of maternal stilbestrol therapy with tumor appearance in young women. *N Engl J Med* 1971;284:878–881.

Herrinton LJ, Weiss NS. Postmenopausal unopposed estrogens: Characteristics of use in relation to the risk of endometrial carcinoma. *Ann Epidemiol* 1993;3:308–318.

Hoover R, Fraumeni JR. Risk of cancer in renal-transplant recipients. *Lancet* 1973;2:55–57.

Hoover R, Glass A, Finkle WD, et al. Conjugated estrogens and breast cancer risk in women. *J Natl Cancer Inst* 1981;67:815–820.

Horwitz RK, Feinstein AR. Alternative analytic methods for case-control studies of estrogens and endometrial cancer. *N Engl J Med* 1978;299:1089–1094.

Jick H, Hunter JR, Dinan BJ, et al. Sedating drugs and automobile accidents leading to hospitalization. *Am J Public Health* 1981;71:1399–1400.

Jick H, Jick SS, Derby LE. Validation of information recorded on general practitioner based computerized data resource in the United Kingdom. *Br Med J* 1991;302:766–768.

Jick H, Walter AM, Watkins RN, et al. Replacement estrogens and breast cancer. *Am J Epidemiol* 1980;112:586–594.

Juurlink DN, Mamdani M, Kopp A, et al. Drug-drug interactions among elderly patients hospitalized for drug toxicity. *JAMA* 2003;289:1652–1658.

Kelly JP, Auquier A, Rzany B, et al. An international collaborative case-control study of severe cutaneous adverse reactions (SCAR): Design and methods. *J Clin Epidemiol* 1995;48:1099–1109.

Kelsey JL, Fisher DB, Holford TR, et al. Exogenous estrogens and other factors in the epidemiology of breast cancer. *J Natl Cancer Inst* 1981;67:327–333.

Kernan WH, Viscoli CM, Brass LM, et al. Phenylpropanolamine and the risk of hemorrhagic stroke. *N Engl J Med* 2000;343:1826–1832.

Koepsell TD, Weiss NS. *Epidemiologic Methods: Studying the Occurrence of Illness.* New York: Oxford; 2003.

Lanier AP, Noller KL, Decker DG, et al. Cancer and stilbestrol: A follow-up of 1,719 persons exposed to estrogens in utero and born 1943–1959. *Mayo Clin Proc* 1973;48:793–799.

Lis Y, Mann RD. The VAMP research multi-purpose database in the U.K. *J Clin Epidemiol* 1995;48:431–443.

Lovastatin Study Group III. A multicenter comparison of lovastatin and cholestyramine therapy for severe primary hypercholesterolemia. *JAMA* 1988;260:359–366.

Maclure M. The case-crossover design: A method for studying transient effects on the risk of acute events. *Am J Epidemiol* 1991;133:144–153.

Mann JI, Inman WHW. Oral contraceptives and death from myocardial infarction. *Br Med J* 1975;2:245–248.

Marks JS, Halpin TJ. Guillain-Barre syndrome in recipients of A/New Jersey influenza vaccine. *JAMA* 1980;243:2490–2494.

Meade TW, Greenberg G, Thompson SG. Progestogens and cardiovascular reactions associated with oral contraceptives and a comparison of the safety of 50- and 30μg oestrogen preparations. *Br Med J* 1980;1157–1161.

Messer J, Reitman D, Sacks HS, et al. Association of adrenocorticosteroid therapy and peptic-ulcer disease. *N Engl J Med* 1983;309:21–24

Miller RR. Drug surveillance utilizing epidemiologic methods: A report from the Boston collaborative Drug Surveillance Program. *Am J Hosp Pharm* 1973;30:584–592.

Mitchell AA, Goldman P, Shapiro S, et al. Drug utilization and reported adverse reactions in hospitalized children. *Am J Epidemiol* 1979;110:196–204.

Murphy TV, Gargiullo PM, Massoudi MS, et al. Intusussception among infants given an oral rotavirus vaccine. *N Engl J Med* 2001;344:564–572.

Myers BD, Ross J, Newton L, et al. Cyclosporine-associated chronin nephropathy. *N Engl J Med* 1984;311:699–729.

O'Meara ES, Rossing MA, Daling JR, et al. Hormone replacement therapy after a diagnosis of breast cancer in relation to recurrence and mortality. *J Natl Cancer Inst* 2001;93:754–762.

Ray WA. Evaluating medication effects outside of clinical trials: New-user designs. *Am J Epidemiol* 2003;158:915–920.

Ray WA, Griffin MR. Use of Medicaid data for pharmacoepidemiology. *Am J Epidemiol* 1989;129:837–849.

Reimer RR, Hoover R, Fraumeni JF, et al. Acute leukemia after alkylating-agent therapy of ovarian cancer. *N Engl J Med* 1977;297:177–181.

Rosenberg L, Mitchell AA, Parsells JL, et al. Lack of relation of oral clefts to diazepam use during pregnancy. *N Engl J Med* 1983;309:1282–1285.

Ross RK, Paganini-Hill A, Gerkins VR, et al. A case-control study of menopausal estrogen therapy and breast cancer. *JAMA* 1980;243:1635–1639.

Schairer C, Lubin J, Troisi R et al. Menopausal estrogen and estrogen-progestin replacement therapy and breast cancer risk (United States). *JAMA* 2000;283:485–491.

Schumacher MC, Jick SS, Jick H, et al. Cimetidine use and gastric cancer. *Epidemiol* 1990;1:251–254.

Selby JV, Friedman GD, Fireman BH. Screening prescription drugs for possible carcinogenicity: Eleven to fifteen years of follow-up. *Cancer Research* 1989;49:5736–5747.

Shiono PH, Mills JL. Oral clefts and diazepam use during pregnancy. *N Engl J Med* 1984;311:919–920.

Silverberg SG, Makowski EL, Roche WD. Endometrial carcinoma in women under 40 years of age. *Cancer* 1977;39:592–598.

Skegg DCG, Doll R. Record linkage for drug monitoring. *J Epidemiol Community Health* 1981;35:25–31.

Skegg DCG, Richards SM, Doll R. Minor tranquilizers and road accidents. *Br Med J* 1979;1:917–919.

Smalley WE, Ray WA, Daugherty JR, et al. Nonsteroidal anti-inflammatory drugs and the incidence of hospitalizations for peptic ulcer disease in elderly persons. *Am J Epidemiol* 1995;141:539–545.

Staffa JA, Chang J, Green L. Cerivastatin and reports of fatal rhabdomyolysis. *N Engl J Med* 2002;346:539–540.

Stanford JL, Weiss NS, Voigt LF, et al. Combined estrogen and progestin hormone replacement therapy in relation to risk of breast cancer in middle-aged women. *JAMA* 1995:274:137–142.

Stern S, Altkorn D, Levinson W. Anticoagulation for atrial fibrillation. *JAMA* 2000;283:2901–2903.

Strand LM, West R. Health databases in Saskatchewan. In Strom BL, ed. *Pharmacoepidemiology*. New York: Churchill Livingstone;1989:189–200.

Thiessen BQ, Wallace SM, Blackburn JL, et al. Increased prescribing of antidepressants subsequent to β-blocker therapy. *Arch Intern Med* 1990;150: 2286–2290.

Venn A, Watson L, Lumley J, et al. Breast and ovarian cancer incidence after infertility and in vitro fertilization. *Lancet* 1995;346:995–1000.

Weinmann S, Glass AG, Weiss NS, et al. Use of diuretics and other antihypertensive medications in relation to the risk of renal cell cancer. *Am J Epidemiol* 1994;140:792–804.

Weiss NS, Sayvetz TA. Incidence of endometrial cancer in relation to the use of oral contraceptives. *N Engl J Med* 1980;302:551–554.

Wysowski DK, Swartz L. Adverse drug event surveillance and drug withdrawals in the United States, 1969–2002. *Arch Intern Med* 2005;165:1363–1369.

Zimmerman HJ, Lewis JH, Ishak KG, et al. Tircynafen-associated hepatic injury: Analysis of 340 cases. *Hepatology* 1984;4:315–323.

7

Natural History of Illness

Studies of the natural history of illness measure health outcomes in persons with a symptom, sign, or condition who are not receiving a therapy that influences the presence or rate of these outcomes.

Natural history studies permit the development of rational strategies for attempting the early detection of untoward consequences in persons who have the symptom, sign, or condition under study. For example, knowledge of the rate at which various early forms of cervical intraepithelial neoplasia progress, either to later forms or to invasive cervical cancer, would have an important bearing on determining the timing of reexamination in women with early intraepithelial neoplasia. Similarly, in patients who have undergone surgery for peptic ulcer disease, the decision to conduct periodic endoscopic surveillance of the gastric remnant, so that early cancer can be identified and treated, depends heavily on these patients' actual incidence of gastric cancer.

Natural history studies also may point to the need for treatment of the condition that is present (and the evaluation of the efficacy of that treatment). For example, it is uncertain how aggressive one should be in treating asymptomatic patients who are discovered to have hypercalcemia on routine examination and who upon further testing are found to have elevated levels of parathyroid hormone but no other apparent cause of hypercalcemia. The results of studies that document subsequent morbidity and mortality in such patients can serve as a guide as to whether parathyroidectomy should be considered or whether it is safe to adopt a conservative approach. As another example, it is necessary to decide whether to place tympanostomy tubes in the ears of children who have bilateral middle ear effusion following acute otitis media. Because children with such effusion show some degree of conductive hearing loss, and because there is reason to believe that conductive hearing loss adversely impairs learning, one might surmise that the presence of bilateral effusion over a number of weeks and months could lead to impaired development of speech and language in children. However, before incurring the hazard and expense associated with the placement of tympanostomy tubes, it would be important to know whether, and to what extent, persistent effusion actually is associated with retardation in the development of speech and language.

With respect to treatment decisions, still another function is served by studies of natural history. For practical reasons, randomized controlled trials and other investigations of therapeutic efficacy cannot be conducted in all segments of the population. Inevitably, to maximize internal validity, these studies of efficacy must employ certain entry criteria that potential subjects must meet, whether those criteria are based on demographic, disease, or other characteristics. You would like to know whether the measurement of treatment efficacy of a given condition obtained in these formal studies pertains to patients who do not meet the entry criteria. Some guidance can be obtained from the results of studies of the natural history of that condition in patients who were not included in the trials. The more similar the natural history in patients who were and were not included, the more likely it is that the results of the treatment trials apply to the latter group.

> *Example:* Randomized controlled trials conducted in hypertensive white and black men have shown antihypertensive therapy to be efficacious in reducing mortality from cardiovascular disease (Collins and Petò, 1994). You have a patient with high blood pressure, a 64-year-old Japanese-American man. Can you expect antihypertensive therapy to be similarly efficacious in him? There have been no studies of the efficacy of antihypertensive therapy similar to the ones cited that were conducted among Japanese American men. So, to begin to answer this question, you turn to studies of natural history—that is, studies that relate mortality from cardiovascular disease to blood pressure level in Japanese men. You find that mortality among Japanese Americans is strongly related to blood pressure (Yano et al., 1984). So it is reasonable to infer that antihypertensive therapy will reduce this patient's risk.

Finally, the results of studies of natural history enable the health care provider to counsel his or her patient by providing a description of possible outcomes that can result from the condition and of the likelihood with which they will occur.

Study Designs for Measuring Natural History

Most commonly, persons with a given symptom, sign, or condition are monitored for the occurrence of the outcome(s) of interest, and the incidence is compared with that in a similarly monitored group of unaffected persons and/or the population as a whole. Cohort (follow-up) studies of this type may either be prospective or retrospective, just as cohort studies that evaluate diagnostic tests or therapy can be. For example, beginning in 1975 the investigators in the Greater Boston Otitis Media Study Group monitored prospectively the occurrence of acute episodes of middle ear disease and the presence of middle ear effusion in a cohort of newborn infants (Teele et al., 1984). The development of speech and language in a sample of these children was then evaluated 3 years later. By way of contrast, investigators at the Kaiser Foundation Health Plan studied the natural history of hypercalcemia using a retrospective approach. In 1976, they identified members who had had at least 2 abnormal calcium values on multiphasic health examinations during the years 1964–1973 (Rubinoff et al., 1983). These patients' medical records were reviewed first to eliminate persons with a "secondary" cause of hypercalcemia and then in the remaining patients to ascertain the occurrence of a wide variety of symptoms and illnesses through 1976.

To determine whether the rate of an outcome in patients with a particular symptom, sign, or condition is atypical, a comparison with the rate in other persons is necessary. The comparison group is often found in the source population from which the affected patients were identified. For example, the development of speech and language at the age of 3 years in the children who often had middle ear effusion was compared with that in children from the same study population who had experienced little or no effusion. The patients with hypercalcemia were compared for subsequent symptoms and illnesses with another group of persons who had normal serum calcium levels during the multiphasic examination.

Alternatively, in some cohort studies of natural history, it is necessary to obtain comparison data from outside the study cohort itself. For example, the rate of subsequent gastric cancer among residents of Olmsted County, Minnesota, who underwent surgery for a peptic ulcer at the Mayo Clinic was compared with that of all Olmsted County residents (Schafer et al., 1983). The analysis and interpretation of studies of this type must consider the possibility that, at the time the initial illness was identified or during the follow-up period, the outcome in question was not sought with the same intensity in the groups being compared (Weiss and Rossing, 1996). For example, let's say you wish to know whether the presence of a ductal in situ carcinoma in one breast predicts the subsequent development of cancer in the contralateral breast. A comparison of the number of women who go on to develop a contralateral cancer with the number expected based on population rates may be hard to interpret, because:

1. At the time a woman is diagnosed as having an in situ tumor in one breast, the other breast would no doubt be thoroughly evaluated for cancer. Only those women with no contralateral tumor at that time would enter a study of the occurrence of subsequent tumors.

Because such screening would not have occurred in most women in the population whose rates are being used for comparison, for a period of time the women with an in situ breast cancer would appear to have a low rate of contralateral disease, whatever their true propensity to develop a second cancer.

2. For some time following a diagnosis of a unilateral in situ breast cancer, there may be closer monitoring of the contralateral breast (e.g., through self-exam, clinical exam, mammography) than would be typical of an unselected woman from the population at large. This would lead to a spuriously high rate of contralateral breast cancer in the cohort of women with in situ tumors.

Because it is almost never possible to quantify these two sources of bias, an effort should be made to minimize them by restricting the analysis of such studies to a period of time somewhat removed from the initial diagnosis, usually 1 or more years. In the contralateral breast cancer example, the time interval omitted should be long enough to allow:

1. The cases in the population at large that were present at the time of initial diagnosis, but not detected due to lack of screening, to have become evident; and
2. The differences in screening intensity between women with and without a history of a unilateral in situ tumor to have lessened or disappeared.

Instead of the *incidence* of a health outcome of concern, some studies measure the *prevalence* of that outcome. For example, in a sample of 295 persons with migraine and 140 other persons, Kruit et al. (2004) administered brain magnetic resonance imaging. They observed 16 (5.4%) of the migraine sufferers to have evidence of a posterior infarct of the brain, in contrast to just 1 (0.7%) of those without migraine. The interpretation of associations observed in studies of this type can be ambiguous: Does migraine predispose to posterior infarction, or does posterior infarction predispose to migraine? In this particular example, the observation of a proportional overrepresentation of posterior locations among incident strokes that occur among patients with migraine (Milhaud et al., 2001) argues in support of the former hypothesis. Nonetheless, a study of stroke incidence in patients with and without migraine would be needed to unequivocally sort out the temporal relation between the 2 conditions (Buring et al., 1995).

It is also possible to undertake case-control studies to evaluate natural history. These case-control studies begin by identifying patients who have sustained the outcome or endpoint of interest. The patients are compared for the presence of earlier symptoms, signs, or conditions with otherwise similar persons who did not sustain this outcome.

Example: Lagergren et al. (1999) identified and interviewed 189 Swedish patients with esophageal adenocarcinoma, approximately 85% of all such patients in that country diagnosed during the years 1995–

1997. Sixty percent reported heartburn or regurgitation at least once per week beginning at least 5 years before diagnosis. In contrast, only 16% of demographically similar controls selected from the Swedish population register reported these symptoms during a comparable period of time (odds ratio = 7.7). Further support of a causal influence of gastroesophageal reflux on the development of esophageal adenocarcinoma comes from: (1) the narrow 95% confidence interval around the observed odds ratio (5.3–11.4); (2) the care taken to *not* include symptoms that may have resulted from the cancer of a nonmalignant antecedent lesion—thus the attention to the period ending 5 years before diagnosis; and (3) in a parallel study, the failure to observe a similar association for squamous-cell carcinoma of the esophagus.

Example: Echocardiographic evaluations were performed in persons under 45 years of age who had sustained an ischemic stroke and in controls of similar age (Gilon et al., 1999). The latter were persons with cancer who had been referred for an assessment of left ventricular systolic function prior to the administration of anthracycline chemotherapy (a treatment associated with reduced contractility), persons in whom the prevalence of mitral valve prolapse might be expected to reflect that in the underlying population. The investigators observed a nearly identical prevalence of mitral valve prolapse in the 2 groups. These results argue that stroke prophylaxis should not be preferentially recommended for persons with mitral valve prolapse.

Case-control studies of natural history do not directly provide the rates of a particular outcome in relation to the presence of a symptom, sign, or condition; in case-control studies, one determines only the frequency of these antecedents in persons who have developed the outcome. Nonetheless, as was seen in Chapter 6, with some additional information on the incidence of the outcome, the data from case-control studies can be used to help estimate these rates.

Issues in the Analysis and Interpretation of Natural History Studies

An Association between a Condition and a Particular Outcome May Not Be Indicative of a Cause-and-Effect Relationship

In the context of natural history studies, the word "cause" means that, if the patient's condition were to be eliminated, his or her chances of developing the untoward outcome would be reduced. It is necessary to reach a verdict of "causal" or "noncausal" for many suspected antecedents of untoward outcomes because usually there will be less interest in detecting or treating the symptom, sign, or condition if it will have no effect on the occurrence of the outcome.

Before concluding that a given condition predisposes a patient to an altered risk of a given outcome, one must at the very least be convinced that the condition *preceded* the outcome and not the other way around. For example, in a number of studies, persons with low levels of serum cholesterol have been noted to experience an increased rate of cancer. Detracting from the hypothesis of a causal relationship between low levels of serum cholesterol and cancer is the suspicion that occult cancer can cause a fall in the serum cholesterol concentration. This suspicion arises from the observation in several (though not all) of these studies that the low cholesterol—cancer association is present for only several years following the cholesterol measurement, but not thereafter (Salmond et al., 1985). Similarly, the 30% increase in all-cause mortality among patients undergoing renal dialysis whose serum cholesterol levels are less than 160 mg/dl, relative to dialysis patients with higher levels, appears not to be due to a harmful effect of a low cholesterol level but rather to the effect of systemic inflammation and malnutrition on both mortality risk and serum cholesterol (Liu et al., 2004).

> *Example:* When conducting their follow-up study of the possible relationship between primary hypogammaglobulinemia and the subsequent occurrence of cancer, Kinlen et al. (1985) wanted to exclude the possibility that such an association could be attributable to immunosuppressive activity of an occult malignancy. Thus they restricted their analysis to cancers that occurred after the first 2 years following diagnosis of hypogammaglobulinemia. Even though this reduced the number of study subjects—61 of the original 377 patients did not survive 2 years—their finding of a fivefold increased cancer risk offers an interpretation that is considerably clearer than it would be had they started to tabulate cancer incidence immediately upon each subject's entry into the study.

Other guidelines used for inferring causal relationships were elaborated on in Chapter 6. Of particular relevance to studies of natural history are the strength of the association and the biologic plausibility of a causal connection between the condition and the outcome. To illustrate the ways in which these guidelines are put to use, let's consider the interpretation of the reports of 2 different studies of natural history.

In the first study, patients with untreated aortic insufficiency were followed and found to have a substantially increased rate of the development of angina, congestive heart failure, and mortality (Spagnuolo et al., 1971). In the second study, during a 5–7 year follow-up, persons over 84 years of age with low systolic or diastolic blood pressure had a substantially increased death rate compared with persons with higher levels of blood pressure (Boshuizen et al., 1998). The question: In patients with aortic insufficiency or in elderly persons with low blood pressure, to what extent would surgical or medical interventions improve on this natural history? The answer: In each instance we must judge first whether the valvular lesion or low blood pressure played a causal role in the development of the untoward outcomes or whether there was some underlying condition that gave rise both to the lesion and to the subsequent events. Although all the patients with aortic insufficiency in the study of Spagnuolo et al. had previously had an attack of rheumatic fever, there has been enough experience with the sequelae of rheumatic fever in the absence of aortic insufficiency to rule out the possibility that the rheumatic fever itself played an important role in the development of angina, heart failure, and so on. On the other hand, a number of chronic illnesses can give rise to hypotension before they prove fatal. Indeed, when the investigators who conducted the study of blood pressure and mortality in the elderly adjusted for indicators of poor health (such as the presence of cardiopulmonary disease or cancer), the increased risk of death seen initially in hypotensive persons disappeared (Boshuizen et al., 1998).

The Relation of the Symptom, Sign, or Condition to the Occurrence of the Outcome May Not Be the Same for All Categories of Patients

Most conditions have a natural history that varies considerably from patient to patient. Some persons with hypertension rapidly develop ocular and renal damage, whereas others seem to suffer no ill effects. Among women with metastatic breast cancer, some are destined to die soon, whereas others may survive for more than a decade.

One of the goals of natural history studies is to predict, among patients with a certain ailment, which ones will do well and which ones will not. To accomplish this goal, it is necessary to monitor the separate natural histories of subgroups of patients defined according to characteristics of the ailment or of the patients themselves.

Example: Patients with unruptured intracranial aneurysms were followed to ascertain the natural history of these lesions (International Study of Unruptured Intracranial Aneurysms Investigators, 2003). Among 1,028 patients with lesions <7 mm in diameter, 7 sustained a ruptured aneurysm during an average of about 4 years of follow-up. Among patients with larger aneurysms, the incidence of rupture was considerably higher and increased steadily in relation to increasing aneurysm diameter. On the basis of these observations, the authors concluded that the risks of mortality and morbidity associated with the presence of small aneurysms (<7 mm) "were often equaled or exceeded by the risks associated with surgical or endovascular repair" and thus that surgical intervention in a patient with a small aneurysm was not warranted. Similarly, after combining the results of 13 cohort studies of persons with abdominal aortic aneurysms, Law et al. (1994) concluded that operative repair only of lesions 6 cm or greater in diameter was warranted. The risk of rupture of a lesion 6 cm or greater (which would be fatal in some 90% of cases) during the following year was estimated to be more than 9%, higher than the anticipated operative mortality of 5%. The risk of rupture of smaller aneurysms was considerably smaller, and so ultrasound monitoring of persons with these lesions, with surgery for those who progressed beyond the 6 cm threshold, was recommended. Indeed, in randomized trials conducted subsequently in patients with abdominal aortic aneurysms < 6 cm in diameter, immediate surgical repair was not associated with any reduction in mortality relative to a strategy of monitoring (Lederle et al., 2002; United Kingdom Small Aneurysms Trial Participants, 2002).

Example: Patients hospitalized with ulcerative colitis during the years 1965–1983 in central Sweden were enumerated from an inpatient registry (Ekbom et al., 1990). With the use of the Swedish National Cancer Registry, the investigators identified cancers subsequently diagnosed in these patients through the end of 1984. Among patients with extensive involvement of the colon (pancolitis), the incidence of colorectal cancer in middle age was nearly 10 times higher in those who were diagnosed as having ulcerative colitis as children than as adults. However, even the latter group developed colorectal cancer 10 times more often than Swedes in general. These data argue that in a patient with pancolitis who is approaching middle age: (a) at a minimum, close medical surveillance for cancer is appropriate no matter when the colitis began; and (b) prophylactic colectomy should be considered seriously if that patient's colitis developed in childhood.

Example: Teele et al. (1984) monitored a cohort of children from birth for the occurrence of otitis media and middle ear effusion and then measured the children's development of speech and language at age 3 years. The duration of middle ear effusion during the first year of life, but not during the next 2 years, was associated with low performance on the speech and language tests. The results of this study and others like it have a direct bearing on the age at which it is deemed appropriate to treat middle ear effusion in children with tympanostomy tubes. (In aggregate, the studies of this question have observed no more than a modest association between middle ear effusion during even the first year of life and preschool language development [Paradise et al., 2000], probably one reason for the failure of randomized trials of the insertion of tympanostomy tubes to document any apparent impact on language proficiency [Paradise et al., 2003].)

Example: The high risk of adverse effects following surgery or radiation therapy for localized prostate cancer has led to efforts to determine which men with this malignancy might have little to gain from these therapies. Chodak et al. (1994) pooled the results of 6 studies of men who were conservatively treated (i.e., they had no surgery or radiation) for localized prostate cancer and found that prognosis was strongly related to the initial tumor grade. Men with Grade 1 or 2 lesions had a 10-year cumulative mortality from prostate cancer of around 13%, whereas the corresponding figure (adjusted for other predictors of survival) was 66% for men with Grade 3 tumors. Although these observations cannot, of course, be used to determine whether surgery or radiation therapy can improve the poor prognosis of patients with a

Grade 3 tumor, they do indicate a subgroup of cases for which the results of conservative therapy leave much to be desired.

Case-control studies of natural history have the capability of delineating subgroups of patients with a given symptom, sign, or condition who are at altered risk of a particular outcome. For example, Dornan et al. (1982) sought to characterize insulin-dependent diabetics who are resistant to the development of retinopathy. They compared 40 persons with long-standing diabetes (average duration 30 years) who had normal eyes with diabetic controls who had retinopathy, matched for duration and age at onset of diabetes, with regard to such characteristics as weight, blood pressure, and smoking habits. (Indirectly, they also attempted to measure the efficacy of hypoglycemic therapy by contrasting the blood glucose levels between the groups during the years following the diagnosis of diabetes.) In a similar way, a case-control study was conducted to determine the factors that predict a "benign" course in multiple sclerosis (Clark et al., 1982).

The Nature of the Study Subjects May Restrict the Generalization of the Observations

When considering to what extent associations found in studies of natural history can be generalized to other patient groups, criteria similar to those espoused earlier for studies of therapy (Chapters 4 and 6) are employed. But to generalize regarding the rate at which subsequent outcomes occur, it is also necessary to take into account the similarity of study and reference populations with regard to the point in the natural history of the condition at which members of the 2 populations are identified. When counseling patients about their prognoses, for instance, you would want to base your appraisal on data from patients "like" them, especially in terms of where they are in the course of the condition. For example, the expected consequences of your patient's hypercalcemia, detected fortuitously from a battery of blood chemistry tests, may differ considerably from those of patients whose hypercalcemia was detected after symptoms (e.g., renal colic) led them to seek medical care.

Example: A study of mortality rates in men with angina pectoris (Frank et al., 1973) was conducted in a large prepaid health care plan. Medical records were reviewed during a 4-year period to identify men aged 25–64 years with symptoms or signs suggestive of angina; these men were asked to attend a special examination. At that time, a detailed history was taken, and from this history a judgment was made as to whether the subject did or did not have angina. Mortality rates in the men with angina were calculated, but these rates would not necessarily apply to men with newly diagnosed angina. The study subjects, being a sample of cases prevalent during a 4-year period, no doubt included a number of cases well along in their natural history, the longevity of whom might be expected to be less than that of new cases. (Mortality rates calculated in this study are less likely to be misleading when used for another purpose—the comparison of subgroups of men with angina to identify those at particularly high or low risk of death.)

Example: The occurrence of a febrile seizure in a child is associated with an increased likelihood of a subsequent nonfebrile seizure. The decision to employ an anticonvulsive medication in a child who has sustained a febrile seizure, given the disorders of behavior and cognition that may accompany such therapy, would be made only if a substantial absolute reduction in the occurrence of subsequent seizures could be achieved. To determine the frequency of seizures following a first febrile seizure, Ellenberg and Nelson (1980) reviewed the results of 26 studies of the question. In 7 of the studies, all children with febrile seizures in a defined population (e.g., a prepaid health care plan, or a large group of children taking part in longitudinal study) were identified; their cumulative incidence of one or more later nonfebrile seizures ranged from 1.5% to 4.6% across the studies. The other 19 studies were of children identified at hospital clinics or referral centers. Those studies observed a much greater incidence of subsequent nonfebrile seizures, ranging from 2.6% to 76.9%. Almost certainly, the studies originating in defined populations are providing information that is most applicable to the typical child who has just sustained a febrile seizure; the results of the clinic-based studies probably were skewed by selective referral of children with characteristics associated with a relatively high risk of nonfebrile seizures.

The Natural History of an Illness May Take a While to Reveal Itself

Serious manifestations of a disease may develop only after a number of years. Thus studies with extended follow-up periods may be necessary to properly document a condition's natural history. For example, important information concerning the natural history of early prostate cancer has been gleaned from a cohort study of 223 men with this condition followed for a mean of 21 years (Johansson et al, 2004). In these men, no tumor-directed therapy was given unless symptomatic progression occurred, at which time orchiectomy or estrogen treatment was administered. Whereas yearly mortality from prostate cancer was between 1.2 and 1.8 per 100 during the first 15 years of follow-up, it rose to 4.4 per 100 after that time (95% confidence interval = 2.2–8.8 per 100). These observations led the authors to conclude that radical treatment of lesions of this type would have its greatest utility in men with a life expectancy that exceeded 15 years.

Questions

7.1. A group of investigators (Gresham et al., 1975) sought to determine "the magnitude and pattern of long-term stroke disability, [to provide] the basis for planning continuing care programs for surviving stroke victims and [to permit] a more accurate prognosis to be made for the individual patient in terms of eventual functional recovery." From the Framingham cohort, a group of more than 5,000 persons monitored for the occurrence of cardiovascular disease since the early 1950s, they identified during the period 1972–1974 the 123 survivors of the 313 persons who had sustained strokes in the prior 20 or so years. They evaluated each subject in terms of his or her functional disability and need for institutional care and compared them in these respects with other living members of the cohort, matched for age and sex. The results were as follows: 31% of the stroke survivors versus 3% of the controls were dependent on others for the activities of daily living; 14% of the stroke survivors versus 2% of the controls were residing in a nursing home or chronic-disease hospital. Did the study accomplish the stated aims of the investigators?

7.2. To test the hypothesis that the presence of endometriosis predisposes women to infertility, a group of investigators conducted a case-control study (Strathy et al., 1982). They reviewed the medical records of 100 women who underwent diagnostic laparoscopy for infertility and, applying the standards of the American Fertility Society, classified 21 as having endometriosis.

The investigators were able to show that a clinical diagnosis of endometriosis was neither a sensitive nor a specific means of determining endometriosis as diagnosed by laparoscopy. Thus the choice of a control group posed a problem, for it was necessary to identify fertile women who had undergone laparoscopy for tubal ligation during the same period. Based on the findings reported in the records of these control subjects, only 4 were deemed to have endometriosis.

a. From these data, can you estimate the risk of infertility in women with endometriosis relative to that in other women? If so, what is that relative risk? If not, why not?

b. Critics of the study claimed that, despite their efforts, the investigators were unable to achieve comparable ascertainment of endometriosis in cases and controls. What do you think was the basis for this criticism?

7.3. In the study of the prevalence of brain infarction (as ascertained by magnetic resonance imaging) among persons with migraine, Kruit et al. (2004) sought to include as participants a representative sample of migraine sufferers in 2 Dutch cities. They screened all 20- to 60-year-old residents of these cities by means of a brief questionnaire. Those who screened as positive were asked to complete a more detailed questionnaire. Among the group of 863 persons who ultimately met the study criteria for the presence of migraine, only 46% previously had been diagnosed with this condition by a physician.

Likely a less expensive way of identifying persons with migraine would have been to review physician records, allowing the investigators to have dispensed with the laborious population survey. What do you believe to be the primary limitation of a study of only diagnosed cases of migraine in trying to determine the prevalence of cerebral infarction in persons with this condition?

Answers

7.1. The study as designed was capable of providing an answer only to the question, Do persons who have survived a stroke have a greater degree of disability than other persons? (It is arguable whether a formal study was needed to provide the obvious answer.) The design left unevaluated the issue of the natural history of stroke that the authors had intended to address. To have done so would have required monitoring survival and functional status in all 313 persons from the time their strokes occurred. This task would have been more difficult than evaluating survivors in 1972–1974, and no doubt information regarding functional status of victims in the 1950s and 1960s would have been imprecise and in some cases unavailable. But such a design would have been responsive to the question the authors had posed.

7.2.a.

		Infertile women	Controls
Endometriosis:	Yes	21	4
	No	79	196

The relative risk can be estimated (by means of the odds ratio) as:

$$(21 \div 79) / (4 \div 196) = 13.0$$

b. The critics might have argued that, with regard to finding endometriosis, laparoscopy done as part of an investigation of a woman's infertility might not be comparable to laparoscopy done to perform a tubal ligation. This especially could be true if (as in this study) no attempt was made to standardize the ascertainment method in cases and controls, which could lead to a substantial overestimation of the risk of infertility associated with endometriosis.

7.3. Among persons with migraine, those who have had this condition diagnosed by a physician may be relatively more severely affected. If migraine severity is related to the prevalence of infarction (for the prevalence of posterior brain infarcts, the data of Kruit et al. (2004) suggest this is so), the restriction of the study population to physician-diagnosed cases of migraine would produce an estimated prevalence of infarction that is spuriously high.

References

Boshuizen HC, Izaks GJ, van Buuren S, et al. Blood pressure and mortality in elderly people aged 85 and older: A community-based study. *Br Med J* 1998;316:1780–1784.

Buring JE, Hebert P, Romero J, et al. Migraine and subsequent risk of stroke in the Physicians' Health Study. *Arch Neurol* 1995;52:129–134.

Chodak GW, Thisbed RA, Gerber GS, et al. Results of conservative management of clinically localized prostate cancer. *N Engl J Med* 1994;330:242–248.

Clark VA, Detels R, Visscher BR, et al. Factors associated with a malignant or benign course of multiple sclerosis. *JAMA* 1982;248:856–860.

Collins R, Petò R. Antihypertensive drug therapy: Effects on stroke and coronary heart disease. In Swales JD, ed. *Textbook of Hypertension.* Oxford, UK: Blackwell Scientific Publications; 1994:1156–1164.

Dornan T, Mann JI, Turner R. Factors protective against retinopathy in insulin-dependent diabetics free of retinopathy for 30 years. *Br Med J* 1982;285:1073–1077.

Ekbom A, Helmick C, Zack M, et al. Ulcerative colitis and colorectal cancer. *N Engl J Med* 1990;323:1228–1233.

Ellenberg JH, Nelson KB. Sample selection and the natural history of disease: Studies of febrile seizures. *JAMA* 1980;243:1337–1340.

Frank CW, Weinblatt E, Shapiro S. Angina pectoris in men: Prognostic significance of selected medical factors. *Circulation* 1973;47:509–517.

Gilon D, Buonanno FS, Jaffe MM, et al. Lack of evidence of an association between mitral-valve prolapse and stroke in young patients. *N Engl J Med* 1999;341:8–13.

Gresham GE, Fitzpatrick TE, Wolf PA, et al. Residual disability in survivors of stroke: The Framingham Study. *N Engl J Med* 1975;293:954–956.

International Study of Unruptured Intracranial Aneurysms Investigators. Unruptured intracranial aneurysms: Natural history, clinical outcome, and risks of surgical and endovascular treatment. *Lancet* 2003;362:103–110.

Johansson J-E, Andren O, Andersson S-O, et al. Natural history of early, localized prostate cancer. *JAMA* 2004;291:2713–2719.

Kinlen LJ, Webster ADB, Bird AG, et al. Prospective study of cancer in patients with hypogammaglobulinaemia. *Lancet* 1985;1:263–266.

Kruit MC, van Buchem MA, Hofman PAM, et al. Migraine as a risk factor for subclinical brain lesions. *JAMA* 2004;291:427–434.

Lagergren J, Bergstrom R, Lindgren A, et al. Symptomatic gastroesophageal reflux as a risk factor for esophogeal adenocarcinoma. *N Engl J Med* 1999;340:825–831.

Law MR, Morris J, Wald NJ. Screening for abdominal aortic aneurysms. *J Med Screening* 1994;1:110–116.

Lederle FA, Wilson SE, Johnson GR, et al. Immediate repair compared with surveillance of small aortic aneurysms. *N Engl J Med* 2002;346:1437–1444.

Liu Y, Coresh J, Eustace JA, et al. Association between cholesterol level and mortality in dialysis patients: Role of inflammation and malnutrition. *JAMA* 2004;291:451–459.

Milhaud D, Bogousslavsky J, VanMelle G, et al. Ischemic stroke and active migraine. *Neurology* 2001;57:1805–1811.

Paradise JL, Dollaghan CA, Campbell TF, et al. Language, speech sound production, and cognition in three-year-old children in relation to otitis media in their first three years of life. *Pediatrics* 2000;105:1119–1130.

Paradise JL, Dollaghan CA, Campbell TF, et al. Otitis media and tympanostomy tube insertion during the first three years of life: Developmental outcomes at the age of four years. *Pediatrics* 2003;112:265–277.

Rubinoff H, McCarthy N, Hiatt RA. Hypercalcemia: Long-term follow-up with matched controls. *J Chron Dis* 1983;36:859–868.

Salmond CE, Beaglehole R, Prior IAM. Are low cholesterol values associated with excess mortality? *Br Med J* 1985;290:422–424.

Schafer LW, Larson DE, Melton J, et al. The risk of gastric carcinoma after surgical treatment for benign ulcer disease. *N Engl J Med* 1983;309:1210–1212.

Spagnuolo M, Kloth H, Taranta A, et al. Natural history of rheumatic aortic regurgitation. *Circulation* 1971;44:368–379.

Strathy JH, Molgaard CA, Coulam CB, et al. Endometriosis and infertility: A laparoscopic study of endometriosis among fertile and infertile women. *Fertil Steril* 1982;38:667–672.

Teele DW, Klein JO, Rosner BA. The Greater Boston Otitis Media Study Group: Otitis media with effusion during the first three years of life and development of speech and language. *Pediatrics* 1984;74:282–287.

United Kingdom Small Aneurysm Trial Participants. Long-term outcomes of immediate repair compared with surveillance of small abdominal aortic aneurysms. *N Engl J Med* 2002;346:1445–1452.

Weiss NS, Rossing MA. Healthy screenee bias in epidemiologic studies of cancer incidence. *Epidemiology* 1996;7:319–322.

Yano K, Reed DM, McGee DL. Ten-year incidence of coronary heart disease in the Honolulu heart program: Relationship to biologic and lifestyle characteristics. *Am J Epidemiol* 1984;199:653–666.

8

Summarizing Evidence

Systematic Reviews and Meta-Analysis

Peter Cummings and Noel S. Weiss

During the 1980s and 1990s, an era in which computerized access to the medical literature became widespread, the systematic review emerged in the medical literature. A systematic review is narrowly focused on a single question or related group of questions. For example, a systematic review might compare laparoscopic hernia repair with open repair in terms of complications, length of time before return to work, and recurrence (Memon et al., 2003). The authors of a systematic review attempt to find all or a clearly described part of the available evidence related to their study questions. They state their strategy for finding the evidence and summarize what they find in tables and text. Many systematic reviews use numerical methods to combine in a quantitative way evidence from relevant studies; this quantitative summary is called "meta-analysis."

By using clearly stated methods to find evidence and combine results, systematic reviews have the potential to maximize objectivity. Decisions about including or excluding evidence may still have a subjective element, but the effect of those decisions can be examined by conducting additional analyses based on different decisions. If the review uses meta-analysis to combine the results of several studies, this generally will enhance statistical power compared with the power in each study alone. This enhanced power may allow the meta-analyst to analyze subgroups of the studied populations. A systematic review or meta-analysis can search for plausible explanations for different findings between studies; as a consequence, the review may produce more than one summary estimate, suggesting that any benefit or harm may vary according to the presence or level of some other factor.

Example: In a series of meta-analyses published from 1982 through 1985, investigators produced evidence suggesting that beta blockers reduce mortality when administered long-term to persons after a myocardial infarction (Lewis, 1982; Lewis and Ellis, 1982; Yusuf et al., 1985). These meta-analyses summarized results regarding 20,312 patients in 23 randomized trials: The pooled odds ratio for death among patients on beta blockers, compared with patients in the control arm of each study, was 0.77 (95% confidence interval = 0.70–0.85). In 1999 a new meta-analysis, including 24,974 patients in 31 trials, reported the same pooled odds ratio of 0.77 (95% confidence interval = 0.69–0.85). (Freemantle et al., 1999).

The conduct of a systematic review can be summarized in the following 8 steps.

Step 1: Finding the Available Evidence

In the United States, the National Library of Medicine has a computerized database (called MEDLINE) of more than 12 million citations to articles in more than 4,800 U.S. medical journals, as well as journals from 70 other countries. An additional 2 million citations are available in OLDMEDLINE. These remarkable databases can be searched through an Internet connection to the National Library's PubMed system (National Center for Biotechnology Information , 2005). Unfortunately, not all evidence is in PubMed. There are several reasons for this: (1) Prior to about 1966, PubMed coverage is incomplete, and prior to 1950 there was no coverage; (2) sometimes articles can be difficult to find due to errors in the indexing or problems with the search strategy; (3) the results of health-related studies do not always appear in biomedical journals. They may be in government agency reports, or in pharmaceutical industry files, or they may simply be unpublished.

Several additional computerized data sources can be searched, such as EMBASE (more representation of European journals), PsycLIT, ERIC (education literature), the Cochrane Library, and others (Bunn et al., 2001). When searching computerized bibliographies, it may be useful to try several combinations of search terms (Lefebvre and Clarke, 2001; Haynes et al., 2005). In addition to computerized data, the bibliographies of textbooks, review articles, and research articles can be examined for relevant information. The final search strategy should be summarized in the systematic review with enough detail so that others could reproduce the search (Moher et al., 1999; Stroup et al., 2000).

Publication Bias

One source of potential bias in any systematic review is the fact that some evidence may not be published. Imagine that we wish to summarize evidence regarding the possibility that treatment A is superior to usual treatment. If in unpublished studies the average size of the association between treatment A and the outcome in question were similar to that in published studies, failure to find the unpublished information would hurt the statistical power of a meta-analysis, but it would not produce bias. But there is evidence that results of studies that suggest no benefit from certain treatments, or even harm, might be less likely to be published than results that do suggest benefit (Dickersin et al., 1987; Dickersin, 1990; Dickersin et al., 1992; Easterbrook et al., 1991; Ioannidis, 1998; Egger et al., 2001; Olson et al., 2002). If this occurs, then the estimate of treatment A effects in the literature will be biased in the direction of greater benefit (or at least less harm). There are several reasons why this type of bias might arise: (1) pharmaceutical companies are not obliged to publish all trials of a drug; they might be more inclined to publish trials whose results are suggestive of benefit (Dickersin and Rennie, 2003); (2) academic investigators who study treatment A might pursue publication only if treatment A appeared to be superior to usual treatment; and (3) some journal editors may be more likely to publish a study if the new treatment appears to be beneficial.

One solution to the possibility of publication bias is to find the unpublished evidence. Unfortunately, it may be difficult or impossible to accomplish this. Recently several major medical journals have taken a step to encourage the registration of randomized trials (DeAngelis et al., 2004; Rennie, 2004). The journal editors have committed themselves not to consider for publication any randomized controlled trial that has not been registered in a publicly available computerized registry prior to enrollment of subjects; the goal is to make sure that trials have been registered before their results are known. It is hoped that this registration procedure will allow a systematic reviewer to find out when results of randomized controlled trials have not been published.

There are concerns about the quality of unpublished data even if such data can be found (Cook et al., 1993; Egger et al., 2001). Unpublished studies may be less methodologically sound than those that are published. Also, in preparation for publication, investigators may devote considerable effort to checking their data and their analyses. In the process of journal review and revision, further checking may correct errors.

Decisions about Study Inclusion

A search for available evidence typically will involve a review of hundreds of article titles, scrutiny of many abstracts, and the reading of dozens of research papers and reports. Decisions about inclusion should be based on a protocol established before the evidence is reviewed and should be independent of the reported study results. The researchers may decide to limit themselves to randomized trials. The focus might be on the effect of treatment A only among children. The review might compare treatment A only with usual treatment or might also compare treatment A with new treatment B.

Step 2. Describing the Evidence Obtained in the Systematic Review

Once the studies to be reviewed have been identified, their characteristics should be summarized in tables that will help investigators and readers see the available evidence. Tables typically include an identifier for each study, such as last name of the first author; the year of publication; characteristics of the study subjects, such as the distribution of age, sex, and severity or type of illness; and study setting. Most important, the tables should present the information used to estimate the association of interest within each study. For example, for a randomized trial it will usually be possible to show the counts of patients in each study arm and the counts of those who had the outcome of interest or summary statistics about the distribution of outcomes if measured on a continuous scale. For nonrandomized studies that estimate associations by means of such measures as an adjusted odds ratio or adjusted rate ratio, it is useful to present the estimate of association for each study, together with information about the statistical variability of that estimate, such as the 95% confidence interval. Often published papers contain enough information to let the reader construct key measures of association and their confidence limits after the fact, even if these measures are not presented in the paper itself.

Meta-analyses typically use numeric summaries of tabular data to estimate associations across all studies or groups of studies. This will not be possible if the authors of the original studies failed to present data that can be summarized: say, counts for 2 × 2 tables or adjusted estimates of association with information about statistical variability. But a systematic review can still summarize the evidence less formally without a meta-analysis. It may be clear from tabular summaries that nearly all the evidence points in one direction or that the available evidence is inconclusive.

Steps 1 and 2 are shared by both systematic reviews and meta-analyses. Systematic reviews typically stop with tabular presentations and discussions that interpret the tabular data. Meta-analysis requires us to move on to the next step.

Step 3. Choosing a Summary Measure of Association

We need to select a statistic that summarizes the association between treatment X and outcome Y. The commonly used statistics fall into 2 groups, ratios and differences. For binary outcomes, such as life or death, commonly used ratio measures include odds ratios, risk ratios, and rate ratios. The risk (or rate) difference also can be used if the outcome is a binary one. If each study subject can experience 2 or more outcome events, such as falls or urinary infections, again rate ratios or rate differences based on total event counts in relation to person-time are useful. If the outcome is continuous, such as blood pressure or cholesterol level, the mean difference may be used.

A Limitation of the Odds Ratio
as a Summary Measure

Odds ratios have desirable statistical properties; for example, they are symmetric, so regardless of how we classify exposure or outcome, the summary odds ratio for exposure will be the inverse of the odds ratio for lack of exposure. When outcomes are uncommon across many studies, the summary odds ratio will closely approximate the summary risk ratio, giving the odds ratio a clear and useful interpretation as a ratio of risks. But when more than about 10% of study subjects have the outcome of interest, the odds ratio will not closely approximate the risk ratio (unless the risk ratio is close to 1). Because an odds ratio that fails to approximate the risk ratio is difficult to interpret, we recommend that odds ratios be avoided as summary measures when outcomes are common (Welch and Koepsell, 1995; Sackett et al., 1996; Altman et al., 1998; Schwartz et al., 1999).

Difficulties When Continuous Outcome Measures
Are on Different Scales

Sometimes the available studies have different measurement scales for the same continuous outcome; for example, different scores for depression, pain, or breathing difficulty. If these scores cannot be translated to a common scale, a pooled meta-analysis is not possible. To create a common scale, the standardized mean difference is sometimes used: the difference in means between the outcome scores of the treatment and control arms divided by the pooled within-group standard deviation over both study arms (or just the control arm) (Hedges and Olkin, 1985; Deeks et al., 2001). This is an effect estimate expressed in standard deviation units for that study. This method assumes that all study populations have the same variability in outcome scores and, therefore, the same standard deviation. Unfortunately, this assumption cannot usually be checked due to the differences in the outcome measurements.

Because study populations may differ both in their response to the treatment and in the amount of variation they have for the study outcome, pooled standardized effect sizes should generally be avoided because: (1) the estimated effect is expressed in standard deviation units, which have no clear clinical interpretation; and (2) between-study differences in standardized treatment effects may be due, in part, to between-study differences in the distribution of outcomes, and, therefore, estimates of heterogeneity, pooled effects, and precision may all be biased (Greenland et al., 1986; Greenland, 1987; Greenland et al., 1991; Cummings, 2004).

Step 4. Choosing a Statistical Method

Details of statistical methods are beyond the scope of this chapter and can be found in many books and articles (Greenland, 1987; Fleiss, 1993; Greenland, 1998; Sutton et al., 2000; Deeks et al., 2001). Here we comment on only a few features of these methods.

Although regression methods for meta-analysis are available (Thompson and Higgins, 2002), stratified methods are most commonly used. There are 2 steps in a stratified analysis: (1) a point estimate of the chosen effect measure and its variance are generated for each study and (2) a weighted average of the point estimate is calculated with an appropriate variance. Stratified methods have some advantages compared with regression: (1) they make the analysis relatively transparent to both the analyst and the reader and (2) the methods generally perform well when outcomes are sparse.

For pooling binary outcomes across studies, the Mantel-Haenszel method for odds ratios and risk ratios is usually an excellent choice; the method works well even when outcomes are sparse in some studies (Mantel and Haenszel, 1959; Greenland and Robins, 1985; Emerson, 1994; Rothman and Greenland, 1998; Deeks et al., 2001; Newman, 2001). To summarize odds ratios, the method of Peto and Yusuf is sometimes used, but in general it offers no advantage over the Mantel-Haenszel method (Yusuf et al., 1985; Emerson, 1994; Deeks et al., 2001). The inverse variance method summarizes the logarithm of study odds ratios or risk ratios using weights that are the inverse of the variance of the logarithm of each study's ratio estimate; this method can be used when the odds ratios or risk ratios for each study are available, along with an estimate of variance, but not the information for the 2×2 tables used to create those ratios (Sutton et al., 2000; Deeks et al., 2001). Inverse variance weights can be applied to continuous outcomes as well.

Step 5. Searching for Differences (Heterogeneity) between Studies

Finding and explaining differences in effect estimates between studies is sometimes more useful than summarizing effects across all studies (Thompson, 1994; Colditz et al., 1995; Greenland, 1998; Thompson, 2001). If treatment A reduced the risk of a bad outcome by 50% in studies of women only (risk ratio 0.5) but doubled the risk of the same bad outcome in studies of men only (risk ratio 2.0), there would be little point in estimating the risk ratio that combines the results for the 2 sexes across all studies. If studies of men only and women only were equally common and similar in size, the summary risk ratio would be about 1.0; this estimate would apply to no one (no patient is half male and half female), and it would obscure the apparent benefit of treatment A for women and the apparent harm for men.

To find differences across studies, a first step is to examine a table or figure of associations, such as risk ratios, with their confidence intervals. The presence of large differences may be easy to detect. To formally test whether the estimates of association from different studies vary more than would be expected by chance, we test the null hypothesis of no difference (homogeneity); a small p value suggests rejection of that hypothesis (Fleiss, 1993; Sutton et al., 2000; Deeks et al., 2001). P values from homogeneity tests depend not only on the size of the differences in effect estimates between studies but also on the number of studies, the size of the study populations, and the frequency of the study outcome. A typical meta-analysis may have fewer than a dozen studies to examine, and in this circumstance tests of heterogeneity are weak; unless the differences are large, the p-value may not be small enough to reject homogeneity even if clinically important heterogeneity is present. A statistic for estimating heterogeneity beyond chance, I^2, has the advantage of being independent of the number of trials (Higgins et al., 2003).

Searching for heterogeneity should not be driven by p values alone. The sources of possible heterogeneity are infinite and include the age and sex distribution of the study populations, differences in study design, differences in the specific form of exposure or intervention, baseline values of key variables (such as serum cholesterol or blood pressure), and length of follow-up. As with any analysis of subgroups, the analysis should be guided, when possible, by knowledge of the subject matter. If, for example, there is reason to believe that the effect of treatment may differ for children and adults, then separate summary estimates of studies of children and studies of adults should be examined. If the results are similar for both age groups, this finding of similarity may contribute useful knowledge.

The source of heterogeneity may be of interest beyond the specific intervention or exposure studied in each investigation. Schulz and colleagues wished to know if some features of randomized trial design were associated with the size of the estimated association reported (Schulz et al., 1995). They examined 250 trials of obstetrical outcomes that were summarized in 33 meta-analyses. All the outcomes were undesirable, and the summary odds ratios from all 33 meta-analyses favored treatment; that is, the odds ratios were less than 1. When trials were not double-blind, the results tended to be particularly favorable toward treatment: The average reported odds ratio for the association between treatment and outcome was 17% lower (95% confidence interval = 4–29) compared with trials that were double-blind. Trials that failed to adequately conceal treatment allocation had an average treatment odds ratio 41% lower (95% confidence interval = 27–52) than the odds ratios for trials with adequate allocation concealment. Through this use of meta-analysis, the investigators identified features of randomized trial design that may be important for obtaining unbiased results.

Quality Scores

More than a dozen quality scoring systems have been published for randomized trials. These different systems assign points to aspects of study design or reporting and sum up these points for a final quality score. Some meta-analysts have used these scores to divide studies into groups based on quality score, to exclude studies based on scores, or to assign different weights to studies based on these scores. However, whereas certain specific items thought to indicate better quality, such as allocation concealment and blinding, may be related to the size of associations observed in randomized trials (Schulz et al., 1995; Jüni et al., 2001a,b), overall quality scores have not been found have this relationship (Emerson et al., 1990; Jüni et al., 1999; Balk et al., 2002). Therefore, quality items should be examined as individual sources of heterogeneity rather than as scores (Greenland, 1994).

Fixed versus Random Effects

The Mantel-Haenszel, Peto-Yusuf, and inverse variance methods all estimate pooled effects using the assumption that the true but unknown association in each study population was the same. These are called "fixed-effects" methods. Differences in the observed associations between studies are attributed to chance variation around a common overall association, due solely to the fact that studies all have finite sample sizes. A fixed-effects summary is an estimate of the impact of the exposure on the average subject across all the studies.

Differences in the size of the association between studies might also arise if there were true heterogeneity among them. There are methods for estimating the overall association, called "random-effects" methods, that assume that the true effects being estimated in each study are a random sample of effects from a fictional population of studies in which the true but unobserved effects fit some hypothetical distribution (such as the normal distribution) (Mosteller and Colditz, 1996). Using this assumption, random-effects methods estimate a between-study variance that is added to the within-study variance of each study (Dersimonian and Laird, 1986; Fleiss, 1993). The pooled association estimated by a random-effects method will tend toward the association found in the average study, not necessarily for the average study participant, as the degree of heterogeneity between studies becomes greater.

Random-effects methods are sometimes described as conservative because the extra between-study variance component should make the confidence interval wider around the pooled estimate. But random-effects summaries weight each study more equally than fixed-effects methods, because the between-study variance is a constant added to each within-study variance. Because of these different weights, the pooled random-effects estimate may be further from an estimate of no effect than the pooled fixed-effects estimate

(Poole and Greenland, 1999; Egger and Smith, 2001); in this sense a random-effects estimate may not be conservative. A study of 21 meta-analyses with evidence of heterogeneity reported that the pooled random-effects risk ratios were more often in the direction of greater apparent treatment effect compared with the fixed-effects risk ratios (Villar et al., 2001). Studies are weighted relatively more equally in a random-effects analysis than in a fixed-effect analysis, and if large studies are, on average, superior in methodological quality to small studies or less prone to publication bias, then random-effects methods may produce estimates that are more biased (Pocock and Hughes, 1990; Greenland, 1994; Poole and Greenland, 1999).

When estimates of the size of the association are similar across studies, the fixed- and random-effects methods will produce the same results. When there is heterogeneity in the observed effect estimates, a pooled estimate across all studies may be unsatisfactory using either method; the fixed-effects assumption of homogeneity is not likely to be true, and the random-effects assumption that the observed estimates are a sample from a hypothetical population may also be implausible. Ideally, the meta-analyst should find the source(s) of the variation and create 2 or more fixed-effects estimates that are derived from homogeneous groups of studies. Nonetheless, there can be practical problems with this approach: (1) the source of heterogeneity may not be apparent; and (2) several sources of heterogeneity may be present, and the choice between these may not be clear. One strategy is to examine both fixed- and random-effects estimates with their confidence intervals (Pocock and Hughes, 1990). This will reveal not only whether there is evidence of heterogeneity but also whether that heterogeneity has much practical influence on point estimates and confidence intervals. If the results are essentially the same with either method, a common situation in practice, fixed-effects results can be reported with the comment that the random-effects analysis produced similar findings. If the results differ importantly and a pooled estimate is still thought to be important (perhaps because the heterogeneity cannot be well explained from the available evidence), it may be reasonable to present both fixed- and random-effects estimates with the caution to readers that neither is wholly satisfactory.

Step 6. Graphical Display of Overall and Study-by-Study Results

Meta-analyses are often accompanied by *forest* plots (Lewis and Clarke, 2001) that show the point estimate of association with confidence intervals for each study, as well as the overall summary estimate and a vertical line that marks the estimate of no effect.

Example: Central venous catheters, often used in seriously ill patients, involve an increased risk of infection. A meta-analysis summarized the incidence of catheter-related bloodstream infection in 11 randomized controlled trials that compared patients given central venous catheters impregnated with antiseptic agents with patients given ordinary central venous catheters (Veenstra et al., 1999). The meta-analysis reported little evidence of heterogeneity ($p = 0.8$) and estimated that the risk of infection was less when antiseptic impregnated catheters were used, compared with ordinary catheters: pooled fixed-effects odds ratio of 0.56 (95% confidence interval = 0.37–0.84). A forest plot of the results is shown in Figure 8.1. The vertical line of no effect corresponds to an odds ratio of 1. The x-axis for the odds ratios is on a log scale. The center of each square marks the odds ratio estimate for that study, and the area of each square is proportional to the weight that study had in the creation of the pooled estimate. The confidence interval for each study is represented by a horizontal line. The pooled estimate and its 95% confidence interval are indicated by the diamond.

Step 7. Sensitivity Analysis

In conducting a meta-analysis, decisions regarding study inclusion, data abstraction, and statistical methods may influence the results. One of the attractive features of a meta-analysis is that the influence of each of these choices can be tested by conducting a sensitivity analysis that makes different decisions (Egger and Smith, 2001; Deeks et al., 2001). For example, suppose that 9 randomized trials had been conducted to address the efficacy of a particular treatment, but in a meta-analysis you decided to exclude 4 of them on the grounds that they had inadequate concealment of treatment allocation prior to subject enrollment. Although it may be reasonable to reject these studies because poor allocation concealment has been reported to be a potential source of bias, it is possible that these studies contained valuable information that might change the overall finding for reasons unrelated to poor allocation concealment. Redoing the analysis with these 4 studies included can be offered as a secondary result. If the findings are essentially unchanged, we can be reassured that the decision to exclude these studies did not influence these findings. If the results are greatly changed, we would have to wonder whether this change is solely due to the poor allocation concealment in the 4 studies or whether it might be related to other differences between those 4 studies and the other 5. Similarly, a sensitivity analysis can check whether different decisions about data extraction or choice of statistical method have much influence on the results. The goal of meta-analysis is to fairly summarize existing evidence; a sensitivity analysis can reveal a fuller picture of this evidence and can reveal the extent to which decisions made by the analyst, which may still have some subjective element, had an influence on the summary picture that emerged.

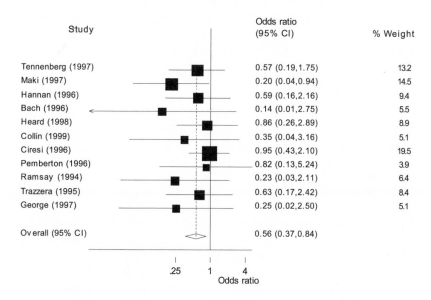

Study		Odds ratio (95% CI)	% Weight
Tennenberg (1997)		0.57 (0.19,1.75)	13.2
Maki (1997)		0.20 (0.04,0.94)	14.5
Hannan (1996)		0.59 (0.16,2.16)	9.4
Bach (1996)		0.14 (0.01,2.75)	5.5
Heard (1998)		0.86 (0.26,2.89)	8.9
Collin (1999)		0.35 (0.04,3.16)	5.1
Ciresi (1996)		0.95 (0.43,2.10)	19.5
Pemberton (1996)		0.82 (0.13,5.24)	3.9
Ramsay (1994)		0.23 (0.03,2.11)	6.4
Trazzera (1995)		0.63 (0.17,2.42)	8.4
George (1997)		0.25 (0.02,2.50)	5.1
Overall (95% CI)		0.56 (0.37,0.84)	

Figure 8.1 Forest plot showing odds ratios for infection among patients given antiseptic impregnated central-venous catheters compared with patients given ordinary central-venous catheters. Each study is identified by last name of first author and publication year. Citations available in Veenstra et al., 1999.

Step 8. Interpretation

A good meta-analysis summarizes current knowledge, but one should not expect that any meta-analysis will settle forever questions about the association of exposure X with outcome Y. Examples of controversial meta-analyses with disputed findings are common (as they are for individual studies). One example is the meta-analyses of the relationship of alcohol consumption to the risk of breast cancer among women. More than half a dozen meta-analyses (Longnecker et al., 1988; Longnecker, 1994; Smith-Warner et al., 1998; Ellison et al., 2001; Hamajima et al., 2002; Shi and Copas, 2004) have been done summarizing evidence from several dozen case-control and cohort studies; although these analyses have reported an elevated risk of breast cancer among women who consume alcohol, the association is weak, and debate continues about whether it represents a causal influence of alcohol.

Controversy is no more or less a feature of meta-analysis than it is for individual studies. We should not expect meta-analyses to be flawless, to be based on perfect studies, or to necessarily settle questions about causation, treatment, or screening. Meta-analysis as a method is arguably superior to narrative reviews that have no defined structure. A good meta-analysis summarizes available evidence. Whether that evidence justifies further research, an end to research on a particular question, or a change in treatment or policy will always be a matter of debate and judgment.

Questions

8.1. In 1991 a meta-analysis reported data from 1,301 patients with acute myocardial infarction in 7 randomized trials and estimated that intravenous magnesium treatment was associated with a reduced risk of death: odds ratio = 0.45 (95% confidence interval = 0.28–0.71) (Teo et al., 1991). In 1992 a large trial of magnesium with 2,316 patients also observed evidence of benefit: risk ratio = 0.76 (95% confidence interval = 0.59–0.99) (Woods et al., 1992). Then, in 1995, a much larger trial of 58,050 patients reported that mortality was slightly *greater* among patients treated with magnesium: risk ratio = 1.055 (95% confidence interval = 0.996–1.117) (ISIS-4 Collaborative Group, 1995).

In a discussion of these and other trials, 2 authors (Borzak and Ridker, 1995) argued that "Probably the most important caveat in interpreting meta-analytic results is that the findings must be considered primarily hypothesis-generating rather than hypothesis-testing. Strong recommendations for treatment should not be made on the basis of even the most promising meta-analysis in the absence of a sufficiently large and well-designed trial."

Do you agree that meta-analyses should only generate hypotheses that should be tested in subsequent large trials?

8.2. Imagine that a well-conducted meta-analysis of treatment A and bad outcome Y reported a risk ratio of 0.6 (95% confidence interval = 0.2–1.9) and the authors concluded: "We found no evidence that treatment A had any effect on outcome Y."

Would you agree? Why or why not?

8.3. Five studies of the possible effect of treatment A on the occurrence of an undesirable binary outcome Y have been published. The risk ratios for Y among the treated compared with the untreated were:

First author	Risk ratio	95% confidence interval
Adams	0.94	0.80–1.10
Brown	0.30	0.09–0.97
Carter	0.98	0.92–1.04
Davis	1.06	0.98–1.15
Evans	1.01	0.92–1.11

A new study has just been completed in which the risk ratio was 0.94 (95% confidence interval = 0.90–0.99). The authors wrote: "Our results were in agreement with those of Brown et al, who reported benefit from treatment A. Four other trials reported no association between treatment and outcome Y." Is this a reasonable summary of the evidence?

Answers

8.1. It should not surprise us that results obtained in a meta-analysis might not always agree with those from later studies. Results might differ for several reasons: (1) both the meta-analysis and a later large trial might be unbiased, but the studies in the meta-analysis and the later large trial differed with respect to some factor that modified the effect of the intervention; (2) the meta-analysis might be biased due to biases in the original studies or because of a bias in the meta-analysis, such as publication bias (Egger and Smith, 1995); (3) the large trial might be biased; or (4) some combination of these problems.

There is some evidence that small trials may be inferior to large trials on average, but other specific reasons for any differences, aside from trial size, can often be identified; these include adequacy of the randomization method, allocation concealment, double blinding, and publication bias (Villar et al., 1995; Flournoy and Olkin, 1995; Cappelleri et al., 1996; Ioannidis et al., 1998; Kjaergard et al., 2001). Nonetheless, when meta-analyses of randomized trials are divided into a single large study and the remaining smaller studies, the results usually agree fairly well (Cappelleri et al., 1996; Kjaergard et al., 2001).

One lesson to be drawn from the magnesium trials is that even large individual studies do not always produce similar results. Findings from the large trial of 2,316 patients did not agree well with those of the very large trial of 58,050 patients.

When do the results of a meta-analysis or a large trial provide sufficient evidence to guide treatment? This will always be a matter of judgment and possible dispute. However, if a systematic summary of prior randomized trials were always considered insufficient until a trial of 58,000 patients were done, most treatment questions would remain forever unresolved. To insist on a large trial, no matter how clear the evidence from well-conducted smaller ones, might result in considerable harm to those in the control arm of the large trial or to those who would forgo the new treatment until that trial was completed.

8.2. The results of the meta-analysis are compatible with both (1) a reduction in the occurrence of Y in persons receiving treatment A and (2) the absence of an effect of A on Y, or even a deleterious effect, plus the play of chance that has led to a suggestion of benefit. Because we cannot distinguish between these alternatives, a claim of "no effect" or "no difference" should be avoided (Altman and Bland, 1995; Alderson and Chalmers, 2003; Alderson, 2004; Altman and Bland, 2004). The authors might have written something like: "Patients who received treatment A had a reduced risk of outcome Y compared with patients who received placebo, but the possible range of effects included both benefit and harm. The clinical utility of treatment A remains uncertain."

8.3. The proposed wording is a form of "vote counting" (Greenland, 1987); it is a summary that ignores the effect estimates and their precision, summarizing results as statistically significant or not. This type of summary is often misleading, as it is here. The new study estimated a risk ratio of 0.94, far from the estimate of 0.30 reported by Brown et al. The only thing the 2 studies have in common is that both had an upper confidence interval bound that was less than 1. The new study estimate of 0.94 was the same as the estimate reported by Adams et al. and fairly similar to the estimates of 0.98, 1.01, and 1.06 reported by 3 other studies. The risk ratio of 0.3 reported by Brown et al. seems unlikely to be correct; it is far below the lower confidence interval boundary of the other 5 studies. A pooled fixed-effects estimate of the risk ratio for all 6 studies (using the inverse variance method) is 0.98 (95% confidence interval = 0.95–1.01). The authors might have written "Pooling our study with the results of 5 previous studies suggests that though treatment A may be beneficial with regard to the incidence of Y, the size of any benefit is probably small."

References

Alderson P. Absence of evidence is not evidence of absence. *BMJ* 2004;328: 476–477.

Alderson P, Chalmers I. Survey of claims of no effect in abstracts of Cochrane reviews. *BMJ* 2003;326:475.

Altman DG, Bland MJ. Absence of evidence is not evidence of absence. *BMJ* 1995;311:485.

Altman D, Bland JM. Confidence intervals illuminate absence of evidence [letter]. *BMJ* 2004;328:1016–1017.

Altman DG, Deeks JJ, Sackett DL. Odds ratios should be avoided when events are common. *BMJ* 1998;317:1318.

Balk EM, Bonis PA, Moskowitz H, et al. Correlation of quality measures with estimates of treatment effect in meta-analyses of randomized controlled trials. *JAMA* 2002;287:2973–2982.

Borzak S, Ridker PM. Discordance between meta-analyses and large-scale randomized, controlled trials: Examples from the management of acute myocardial infarction. *Ann Intern Med* 1995;123:873–877.

Bunn F, DiGuiseppi CG, Roberts I. Systematic reviews of injury studies. In Rivara FP, Cummings P, Koepsell TD, et al., eds. *Injury Control: A Guide to Research and Program Evaluation.* New York: Cambridge University Press; 2001:183–195.

Cappelleri JC, Ioannidis JPA, Schmid CH, et al. Large trials vs meta-analysis of smaller trials: How do their results compare? *JAMA* 1996;276:1332–1338.

Colditz GA, Burdick E, Mosteller F. Heterogeneity in meta-analysis of data from epidemiologic studies: A commentary. *Am J Epidemiol* 1995;142: 371–382.

Cook DJ, Guyatt GH, Ryan G, et al. Should unpublished data be included in meta-analyses? Current convictions and controversies. *JAMA* 1993;269: 2749–2753.

Cummings P. Meta-analysis based on standardized effects is unreliable [editorial]. *Arch Pediatr Adolesc Med* 2004;158:595–597.

DeAngelis CD, Drazen JM, Frizelle FA, et al. Clinical trial registration: A statement from the International Committee of Medical Journal Editors. *JAMA* 2004;292:1363–1364.

Deeks JJ, Altman DG, Bradburn MJ. Statistical methods for examining heterogeneity and combining results from several studies in meta-analysis. In Egger M, Smith GD, Altman DG, eds. *Systematic Reviews in Health Care: Meta-analysis in Context.* London: BMJ Publishing Group; 2001:285–312.

Der Simonian R, Laird N. Meta-analysis in clinical trials. *Cont Clin Trials* 1986;7:177–188.

Dickersin K. The existence of publication bias and risk factors for its occurrence. *JAMA* 1990;263:1385–1389.

Dickersin K, Chan S, Chalmers TC, et al. Publication bias and clinical trials. *Control Clin Trials* 1987;8:343–353.

Dickersin K, Min YI, Meinert CL. Factors influencing publication of research results: Follow-up of applications submitted to two institutional review boards. *JAMA* 1992;267:374–378.

Dickersin K, Rennie D. Registering clinical trials. *JAMA* 2003;290:516–523.

Easterbrook PJ, Berlin JA, Gopalan R, et al. Publication bias in clinical research. *Lancet* 1991;337:867–872.

Egger M, Smith GD. Misleading meta-analysis. *BMJ* 1995;310:752–754.

Egger M, Smith GD. Principles of and procedures for systematic reviews. In Egger M, Smith GD, Altman DG, eds. *Systematic Reviews in Health Care: Meta-analysis in Context.* London: BMJ Publishing Group; 2001:23–42.

Egger M, Dickersin K, Smith GD. Problems and limitations in conducting systematic reviews. In Egger M, Smith GD, Altman DG, eds. *Systematic Reviews in Health Care: Meta-analysis in Context.* London: BMJ Publishing Group; 2001:43–68.

Ellison RC, Zhang Y, McLennan CE, et al. Exploring the relation of alcohol consumption to risk of breast cancer. *Am J Epidemiol* 2001;154:740–747.

Emerson JD. Combining estimates of the odds ratio: The state of the art. *Stat Methods Med Res* 1994;3:157–178.

Emerson JD, Burdick E, Hoaglin DC, et al. An empirical study of the possible relation of treatment differences to quality scores in controlled randomized clinical trials. *Control Clin Trials* 1990;11:339–352.

Fleiss JL. The statistical basis of meta-analysis. *Stat Meth Med Res* 1993;2: 121–145.

Flournoy N, Olkin I. Do small trials square with large ones? *Lancet* 1995;345: 741–742.

Freemantle N, Cleland J, Young P, et al. Beta blockade after myocardial infarction: Systematic review and meta regression analysis. *BMJ* 1999;318: 1730–1737.

Greenland S. Quantitative methods in the review of epidemiologic literature. *Epidemiol Rev* 1987;9:1–30.

Greenland S. Invited commentary: A critical look at some popular meta-analytic methods. *Am J Epidemiol* 1994;140:290–296.

Greenland S. Meta-analysis. In Rothman KJ, Greenland S, eds. *Modern Epidemiology*. Philadelphia: Lippincott-Raven; 1998:643–673.

Greenland S, Maclure M, Schlesselman JJ, et al. Standardized regression coefficients: A further critique and review of some alternatives. *Epidemiology* 1991;2:387–392.

Greenland S, Robins JM. Estimation of a common effect parameter from sparse follow-up data. *Biometrics* 1985;41:55–68.

Greenland S, Schlesselman JJ, Criqui MH. The fallacy of employing standardized regression coefficients and correlations as measures of effect. *Am J Epidemiol* 1986;123:203–208.

Hamajima N, Hirose K, Tajima K, et al. Alcohol, tobacco and breast cancer: Collaborative reanalysis of individual data from 53 epidemiological studies, including 58,515 women with breast cancer and 95,067 women without the disease. *Br J Cancer* 2002;87:1234–1245.

Haynes RB, McKibbon KA, Wilczynski NL, et al. Optimal search strategies for retrieving scientifically strong studies of treatment from Medline: Analytical survey. *BMJ* 2005;330:1179.

Hedges LV, Olkin I. *Statistical Methods for Meta-Analysis*. San Diego, CA: Academic Press; 1985.

Higgins JP, Thompson SG, Deeks JJ, et al. Measuring inconsistency in meta-analyses. *BMJ* 2003;327:557–560.

Ioannidis JP. Effect of the statistical significance of results on the time to completion and publication of randomized efficacy trials. *JAMA* 1998;279:281–286.

Ioannidis JPA, Cappelleri JC, Lau J. Issues in comparisons between meta-analyses and large trials. *JAMA* 1998;279:1089–1093.

ISIS-4 (Fourth International Study of Infarct Survival) Collaborative Group. ISIS-4: A randomised factorial trial assessing early oral captopril, oral mononitrate, and intravenous magnesium sulphate in 58,050 patients with suspected acute myocardial infarction. *Lancet* 1995;345:669–685.

Jüni P, Altman DG, Egger M. Assessing the quality of randomised controlled trials. In Egger M, Smith GD, Altman DG, eds. *Systematic Reviews in Health Care: Meta-analysis in Context*. London: BMJ Publishing Group; 2001a:87–108.

Jüni P, Altman DG, Egger M. Systematic reviews in health care: Assessing the quality of controlled clinical trials. *BMJ* 2001b;323:42–46.

Jüni P, Witschi A, Bloch R, et al. The hazards of scoring the quality of clinical trials for meta-analysis. *JAMA* 1999;282:1054–1060.

Kjaergard LL, Villumsen J, Gluud C. Reported methodologic quality and discrepancies between large and small randomized trials in meta-analyses. *Ann Intern Med* 2001;135:982–989.

Lefebvre C, Clarke MJ. Identifying randomised trials. In Egger M, Smith GD, Altman DG, eds. *Systematic Reviews in Health Care: Meta-analysis in Context*. London: BMJ Publishing Group; 2001:69–86.

Lewis JA. ß-blockade after myocardial infarction: A statistical view. *Br J Clin Pharmacol* 1982;14:15S-21S.

Lewis JA, Ellis SH. A statistical appraisal of post-infarction beta-blocker trials. *Primary Cardiol* 1982;8:31–37.

Lewis S, Clarke M. Forest plots: Trying to see the wood and the trees. *BMJ* 2001;322:1479–1480.

Longnecker MP. Alcoholic beverage consumption in relation to risk of breast cancer: Meta-analysis and review. *Cancer Causes Control* 1994;5:73–82.

Longnecker MP, Berlin JA, Orza MJ, et al. A meta-analysis of alcohol consumption in relation to risk of breast cancer. *JAMA* 1988;260:652–656.

Mantel N, Haenszel W. Statistical aspects of the analysis of data from retrospective studies. *J Natl Cancer Inst* 1959;22:719–748.

Memon MA, Cooper NJ, Memon B, et al. Meta-analysis of randomized clinical trials comparing open and laparoscopic inguinal hernia repair. *Br J Surg* 2003;90:1479–1492.

Moher D, Cook DJ, Eastwood S, et al. Improving the quality of reports of meta-analyses of randomised controlled trials: The QUOROM statement. Quality of Reporting of Meta-analyses. *Lancet* 1999;354:1896–1900.

Mosteller F, Colditz GA. Understanding research synthesis (meta-analysis). *Annu Rev Public Health* 1996;17:1–23.

National Center for Biotechnology Information. PubMed Overview. Available at: *http://www.ncbi.nlm.nih.gov/entrez/query/static/overview.html#Database%20Coverage*. Accessed June 12, 2005.

Newman SC. *Biostatistical Methods in Epidemiology.* New York: John Wiley & Sons; 2001.

Olson CM, Rennie D, Cook D, et al. Publication bias in editorial decision making. *JAMA* 2002;287:2825–2828.

Pocock SJ, Hughes MD. Estimation issues in clinical trials and overviews. *Stat Med* 1990;9:657–671.

Poole C, Greenland S. Random-effects meta-analyses are not always conservative. *Am J Epidemiol* 1999;150:469–475.

Rennie D. Trial registration: A great idea switches from ignored to irresistible. *JAMA* 2004;292:1359–1362.

Rothman KJ, Greenland S. *Modern Epidemiology.* Philadelphia: Lippincott-Raven; 1998.

Sackett DL, Deeks JJ, Altman DG. Down with odds ratios! *Evid Based Med* 1996;1:164–166.

Schulz KF, Chalmers I, Hayes RJ, et al. Empirical evidence of bias: Dimensions of methodological quality associated with estimates of treatment effects in controlled trials. *JAMA* 1995;273:408–412.

Schwartz LM, Woloshin S, Welch HG. Misunderstanding about the effects of race and sex on physicians' referrals for cardiac catheterization. *N Engl J Med* 1999;341:279–283.

Shi JQ, Copas JB. Meta-analysis for trend estimation. *Stat Med* 2004;23:3–19.

Smith-Warner SA, Spiegelman D, Yaun SS, et al. Alcohol and breast cancer in women: a pooled analysis of cohort studies. *JAMA* 1998;279:535–540.

Stroup DF, Berlin JA, Morton SC, et al. Meta-analysis of observational studies in epidemiology: A proposal for reporting. *JAMA* 2000;283:2008–2012.

Sutton AJ, Abrams KR, Jones DR, et al. *Methods for Meta-analysis in Medical Research.* Chichester, England: John Wiley & Sons; 2000.

Teo KK, Yusuf S, Collins R, et al. Effects of intravenous magnesium in suspected acute myocardial infarction: Overview of randomised trials. *BMJ* 1991;303:1499–1503.

Thompson SG. Why sources of heterogeneity in meta-analysis should be investigated. *BMJ* 1994;309:1351–1355.

Thompson SG. Why and how sources of heterogeneity should be investigated. In Egger M, Smith GD, Altman DG, eds. *Systematic Reviews in Health Care: Meta-analysis in Context.* London: BMJ Publishing Group; 2001:157–175.

Thompson SG, Higgins JP. How should meta-regression analyses be undertaken and interpreted? *Stat Med* 2002;21:1559–1573.

Veenstra DL, Saint S, Saha S, et al. Efficacy of antiseptic-impregnated central venous catheters in preventing catheter-related bloodstream infection: A meta-analysis. *JAMA* 1999;281:261–267.

Villar J, Carroli G, Belizan JM. Predictive ability of meta-analyses of randomised controlled trials. *Lancet* 1995;345:772–776.

Villar J, Mackey ME, Carroli G, et al. Meta-analyses in systematic reviews of randomized controlled trials in perinatal medicine: Comparison of fixed and random effects models. *Stat Med* 2001;20:3635–3647.

Welch HG, Koepsell TD. Insurance and the risk of ruptured appendix [letter]. *N Engl J Med* 1995;332:396–397.

Woods KL, Fletcher S, Roffe C, et al. Intravenous magnesium sulphate in suspected acute myocardial infarction: Results of the second Leicester Intravenous Magnesium Intervention Trial (LIMIT-2). *Lancet* 1992;339:1553–1558.

Yusuf S, Peto R, Lewis J, et al. Beta blockade during and after myocardial infarction: An overview of the randomized trials. *Prog Cardio Dis* 1985;27:335–371.

Index